The Truth About Building Muscle

Fat Loss Edition

By: Jeffrey Bedeaux

Table of Contents

Eat well and often

Combine machines and free weights

Keep a daily workout record

Diet to obtain muscular definition and low bodyfat

Questions and answers

Terms and definitions

Introduction

About this book

Hello and welcome! Thanks for purchasing my new e-book. It's loaded with revolutionary proven knowledge and techniques that will allow you to quickly and efficiently transform your body to whatever level of fitness and muscularity you desire. You can do muscle toning or firming or conditioning for a sport or **even adding 20, 40, 60 pounds of new, hard muscle** to your frame. All without drugs and without spending a fortune on nutritional supplements and without wasting your time in the gym.

You see, a while ago my 25-year-old friend told me was getting into lifting weights at the gym and he wanted to know what I thought he should be doing in the gym to maximize his results. He knew that I wrote books on the subject, performed research on trainees from 16 to 82 years of age, measured the results every step of the way and synthesized them into full workouts and specialization workouts. He knew all that and more but he didn't want to read that much, he just wanted his best friend to tell him the core knowledge from all those books and all that research. The best of the best without any preamble, padding myself on the back or self-serving BS about how smart I was compared to others. So I gave it to him. Nothing more; nothing less.

That made me realize I really could condense what I've learned developing new data, feedback from customers, and experience from personal consultations. Everything into a book that I could make available to anyone in the world via the Internet.

And that's what you have right now. The best information garnered from years of research in real world testing. I urge you to read every word of it. The knowledge you need is in these pages and is laid out in a concise format and I don't repeat the same things over and over. That is with the exception of safety. Safety is the most important piece of information you can get out of this book. With that said I wouldn't dwell on it too much.

<u>**Getting the most from this book**</u>

If you are like most guys, you're tempted to turn to the chapters on workouts and dive right into your workouts with those killer techniques and principles. That's because most muscleheads see bodybuilding as merely hoisting weights up-and-down, over and over, slowly increasing the weight, under some misguided concept of this is what builds muscle. These are the guys who are always on the look out for the magic routine that has eluded them for so long. Don't make that mistake!

Now I know you're not going to like to hear this, but read this manual all the way through before beginning your program. I want you to get on the gym floor in the quickest time possible but I want you to be armed with the advanced knowledge needed to put that time to good use. If you skip a chapter thinking you already know everything needed to know about that training factor, you could be setting yourself up for a big disappointment. But don't worry I'll be there every step of the way.

We will be covering a lot of information in this book. Information that is anything but common knowledge even among the professional bodybuilders who rely on anabolic steroids for their massive gains. Well, there you have it. I've sufficiently warned you of the dangers of skipping ahead in this book and I've given you a couple of "extra emphasis" tools to make sure you get the most important details from all information I have jammed into these pages.

Also, you will notice a couple of inches of open space at the bottom of each page; I did this for a reason. I want you to write down and highlight the most important parts for you. This open space is for your notes. By reading and writing the ideas that really connect with you, you will be able to absorb and use those points without even being aware of it. Print out this book and write all over it; I want you to squeeze every benefit out of the huge amount of information within these pages.

Two other tools you will see throughout this book that will help you understand the key points are *The Doctor Says* dialog box and the *Doctor's Prescription* dialog box. Look for boxes like these as you are reading:

<table>
<tr><td>The Doctor Says:
"Look here for insights into the topic being discussed."</td></tr>
</table>

<table>
<tr><td>Doctor's Prescription:
Look in these boxes for action steps you can take.</td></tr>
</table>

These 2 dialog boxes will help you get the most important information first. Also use them as a guideline for writing your own notes at the bottom of each page. After you have read this book you can skim through it later and read only the dialog boxes and your personal notes to re-connect with all the information contained in this book. I have found this technique to be very valuable to me when I want to skim a book I have already read and review the key points.

So here's what I want you to do now. If you have already been busting your ass in the gym training three to four days or more per week. Take a week off! You'll understand why later, but for now just plan on using that week to review this manual and fully prepare for your fiery return. If you're relatively new to bodybuilding, or it has been awhile since you've been in the gym, take the next week to introduce your body to what it's about to experience. In order to avoid overloading your body to the point of shutdown it's wise to begin a light exercise routine to prepare your muscles, joints and ligaments for the upcoming barrage. You don't want to go all out to the point you can barely move the next day. That would defeat the whole purpose of the first couple weeks of this program. Besides if you're looking for is an intense workout session, the real workout is coming up.

Dedication

This book is dedicated to every bodybuilder and athlete who has an acquiring rational mind; to every person who can throw off the chains of comfortable habit and unproven premises and move into new direction that is guided by reason and observational evidence, no matter where that direction takes him; to every person to try something immediately and thinks "How can I make this better?" To every person who is unafraid to challenge the false beliefs of the herd and lead others out of the cave and into the light.

In the world of bodybuilding it is these people with these genetics who are truly the greatest champions of the human race. To these people not just in the science of human strength but also in every science we all owe our enormous gratitude.

<u>Why an e-book?</u>

Some people ask me why I wrote this as an e-book. I could have written the draft of this book and taken to a mainstream book publisher, but there are a few reasons why I self published this as an e-book and they all benefit you.

Freedom of content: E-books can contain links to related material, special pages or even built-in programs. Also big publishing companies don't like controversy. They don't like writers being too blunt about certain topics. They prefer to re-edit or re-word certain things. With an e-book, which I both write and publish, I conclude whatever content I want to include. Which leads me to…

Freedom of style: Any writer does better when he uses his own "voice". For example, in a mainstream publication I would have to say, "many professional bodybuilders use dangerous drugs to augment their muscular development." But in my own e-book I can say, "pro bodybuilding is filled with unbridled use of every type of drug imaginable.

Steroids represent less than 10 percent of what drugs bodybuilders actually use today. The full truth is that they use up to 20 prescription drugs at the same time and 1000% of the recommended safe dose. They take drugs intended for diabetes, cancer, dwarfism, pain, bloating, cardiology, hematology, impotence; the list goes on and on.

Athletes and regular folks are dropping dead every year and the huge meltdown is coming because the real health effects (tumors, heart failure, kidney failure, etc) appear to take at least fifteen years to show up. Soon we'll be hearing about the failing health of the great names of bodybuilding from the '80s and '90s, if you haven't heard already." Try finding that kind of plain talk in a nice mainstream book. I'm sure you won't find it especially if the author puts down supplements anyway since that's where the real cash cow is in bodybuilding.

Freedom from templates: Mainstream publishers have a formula they have to follow. It is just the realities of the book business. Right now is the larger book format (9" x 11") with approximately 220 pages; it is all about shelf space in the bookstores and perceived value. So a new e-book with about 120 pages loaded with new ideas that's guaranteed to put 40 pounds of muscle on you doesn't have a prayer of getting into print, but a 220 page book showing women doing "workouts" with 3 pound dumbbells gets in every bookstore and featured every woman's magazine.

The perception of what is valuable is very different from what really has value in the gym. An e-book format allows me to get right to the point without adding a bunch of filler, such as lots and lots of pictures that you have already seen, to get the book up to 220 pages.

The amount of information packed into this e-book took 17 years to determine and compile. It can unlock the greatest muscle growth you've ever experienced. When Einstein writes $E=MC^2$ on a piece of paper, it doesn't take a many pages but that knowledge can unlock enormous power.

Freedom of marketing: Digital content and the Internet is the wave of the future in publishing. When a mainstream book is published it gets an initial marketing push by the publisher and then it's all done. E-books can be promoted by links, banners, affiliate programs, and "word of mouse" that keep it in front of bodybuilders every day. Why should you care about that? The financial success of this e-book fuels the next one and that brings you more useful research information instead of the crap that's available in many books. As you can see in the bookstores, mainstream publishers say the same thing day after day, year after year.

Freedom of access: Less than 5% of the world's population lives in America. It can be pretty difficult and expensive to get an American book delivered to Turkey. But an e-book can be delivered around the world without extra costs and you can be reading it 20 seconds after you buy it.

And I'm not talking hypothetically here; this e-book not only sold copies in the United States and Canada, it also sold in the United Kingdom, France, Germany, Sweden, Switzerland, Australia, Brazil, Ireland, Singapore, South Africa, Denmark, Malaysia, China, Japan, Belarus, American Samoa and the Netherlands. All in the first 60 days!

Like the bodybuilders in the above countries around the world you're about to discover this e-book is absolutely loaded with useful information you can apply in your next workout. You're literally minutes away from the most productive workouts of your life.

<u>Why I wrote this book</u>

First let me explain why I wrote this book, I'll phrase it into a short story were I'm sure you can identify with the main character.

Let me introduce you to Average Joe. Joe is very typical of the bodybuilders trying to pack on muscle in today's gyms. Determined to look like "the huge guys" in the magazines, he signed up for his membership at the local gym, buys his weightlifting gloves and belt and all the other "essential tools" for packing on the pounds, and begins his quest.

At the gym he follows the lead of all the other "muscleheads" and begins bench pressing, curling, and squatting the most weight he can. Like the other misinformed Joes, he thinks that working harder and harder, steadily increasing the weight on the bar will force his body into growth beyond his wildest dreams. He makes some gains; enough to keep pushing on but soon finds himself stagnated.

Not seeing any more strength or size development Joe decides to go to the next level. He looks around the gym for the biggest iron pumping "consultant" he can find that also looks friendly enough to talk to. That guy is The Juice. Joe approaches Juice to inquire about the secrets to his bodybuilding. Juice tells Joe everything he knows about what exercises to choose, how much weight to use, what to eat and what "super supplements" to use.

Joe sets out again following everything Juice tells him; positive he now has the missing links to maximum growth. Some of what Juice told Joe was enough to move him out of his plateau temporarily. Within a few weeks he finds his strength and size stalemated again.

Frustrated Joe decides to turn to the "experts". He goes to the local bookstore and picks up every bodybuilding magazine they have and begins his research. Obviously with arms and legs the size of telephone poles and a chest the size of 2 Webster's dictionaries, anything these pros have to say must be gospel. Then there all the ads for the top-secret supplement discoveries promising you God-like powers from all the "latest" scientific research.

Confused and frustrated Joe spent a small fortune on supplements and is back in the gym. He is loaded with tips from all the pros and has so many "secret potions" running through his veins that he can be declared off-limits as a toxic waste dump! He makes a small gain, only to find it whither away as he hits "the wall". The wall is the place that all beginning and novice bodybuilders hit when they realize that building muscle is a whole lot harder than those hulking professionals in the magazines make it look.

Now comes the moment of truth. Here are the facts.

Fact: All those pro bodybuilders trying to coax you to purchase the next wave of natural supplements guaranteeing massive growth, got that big not from the natural supplements they are marketing but rather by pumping massive quantities of anabolic steroids into their veins.

Fact: The killer pre-contest and mass building routines those pros let you in on are enough to throw any bodybuilder into chronic overtraining without the aid of a serious dose of dangerous growth hormone and steroids. Or make you sick from a depressed immune system or seriously injure yourself.

Fact: The bodybuilding supplement market is a multi-multi-million dollar industry that is supported by well-intentioned serious seekers of muscle and fitness such as yourself, fall prey to the ads and articles designed for one thing, to take your hard earned money.

Fact: Supplement manufacturers and gym owners all follow the six-month rule of marketing. Basically six months is how long research has shown it takes the average "seeker of strength" to join a gym, purchase the supplements they're convinced they need, reach the wall where they see no more gains, get frustrated, and quit their workout program.

Fact: Those same bodybuilding magazines that projected air of "objectivity" actually own many of the supplements they're advertising and are recommending in their magazines.

Here are some of the worst offenders:

Flex — Weider Supplements
Muscle & Fitness — Weider Supplements
MuscleMag — Muscle Tech
Muscular Development — Twinlab
Muscle Media — EAS

These companies weren't stupid. They realized early on that they could sell you a magazine full of great looking perfectly sculpted columns of muscle to make you feel puny and weak; then offer you ad after ad of expensive supplements with pumped up scientific claims to milk you for even more of your dough.

<u>Be careful</u>

Caution: This program involves a systemic progression of muscular overload that leads to lifting extremely heavy weights. As a result, a proper warm-up of muscles, tendons, ligaments, and joints is mandatory at beginning of every workout.

Warning: As this is a very intense program, it requires both a thorough knowledge of proper exercise form and a base level of strength fitness. Although exercise is very beneficial, the potential does exist for injury, especially if the trainee is not in good physical condition. As always consult with your physician before beginning any program of progressive weight training or exercise. If you feel any strain or pain when you start exercising, stop immediately and consult your physician.

Lose fat

Eating to lose body fat

One pound of body fat contains about 3,500 stored calories. You must reduce your caloric intake by 3,500 calories a week to lose one pound per week or increase your activity level to burn 3,500 extra calories per week. **You must either eat fewer calories or burn more calories by increasing your activity level or a combination of both—it's that simple.**

But don't expect getting lean, ripped, or shredded to be so easy. The first few days on a diet, you may lose several pounds. That's because your body takes the easy way out when it needs energy. It uses up your stored carbohydrate (glycogen). Carbohydrates contain a relatively large amount of water. When you begin a diet, you can lose a lot of fluid, but no fat. You have a weight loss that only lasts until your next drink of water.

Your body does other things to preserve body fat. When it has used up its carbohydrate stores, it will shift your metabolism into a slower rate. You will discover you are moving more slowly and have less energy because you have used up your carbohydrate (quick energy) stores. **Our bodies have been conditioned, over time, to guard against famine and will do almost anything to conserve fat.** If weight loss is not done properly, too much precious muscle mass will be lost. But, if you are persistent, as a last resort, your body will begin to use its fat stores for energy.

Don't look too long for easy answers when trying to lose body fat. You are going to have to pay a price if you are truly committed to getting lean. There are no fancy pain-free diets or state-of-the-art supplements that are going to do the bulk of the work for you. Don't try to fool yourself. Or you will set yourself up for failure and disappointment.

> The Doctor Says:
> There are only 3 major ways to lose weight (preferably bodyfat). Eat less calories, burn more calories or a combination of the two.

If you want to lose excess body fat, the bottom line is you have to eat fewer calories than you burn each day. There are several ways to burn more calories than you eat. You can add more cardiovascular work to your training regimen. You can also simply eat less food throughout the day. You can even do a combination of these two strategies by doing more cardiovascular training and eating less food.

How quickly you will shred that body fat will depend on how much of a deficit you create between the calories you consume and the calories you burn on a daily basis. And for how long you wish to go through the sacrifice and pain it takes to train and/or diet this way.

Although my advice doesn't make the fat loss process a whole lot easier, it should make the process simpler. Without being distracted by constantly searching for unrealistic, quick fix solutions, or super supplements. You can now focus on the task in front of you, get to work and achieve the results you truly desire.

Here is an example breakdown of how a 200 pound bodybuilder can gain/maintain muscle while dropping bodyfat. It will give you 300 grams of carbs and 200 grams of protein.

Meal one: Breakfast
75-100 grams of carbs
35 grams of protein

Meal two: Mid-morning snack
25 grams of carbs
25 grams of protein

Meal three: Lunch
50 grams of carbs
35 grams of protein

Meal four: Postworkout
75-100 grams of carbs
55 grams of protein

Meal five: Dinner
50 grams of carbs
35 grams of protein

Meal six: Bedtime snack
No carbs
25 grams of protein

There's no substitute for hard work when it comes to losing fat

When it comes to dieting to lose bodyfat, there's no substitute for hard work. Believe me, I really wish this were not the case. If it really was that easy then everyone would have already done it and we would live in a world of perfect bodies! Unfortunately, however, you must burn more calories than you ingest every day to lose that stubborn body fat.

Low-fat diets, high fat diets, carefully watching your fat intake, or paying close attention to the glycemic index in your foods, it doesn't matter. When the day is done, you must burn more calories than you eat. It doesn't even matter if all the food you eat is healthy, non-junk food, or "clean," its total must be lower than your maintenance level.

As the saying goes, "God puts a price-tag on everything." If you've accumulated some body fat and desperately want to get rid of it, you are going to have to pay the price. The price may be spending more time sweating on a treadmill, feeling hungry on occasion, or both. Whatever method you choose, there will be some pain involved. I would be lying to you if I told you any differently.

Anyone who tells you differently is just flat-out misleading you! I firmly believe it is our desire to discover some painless alternative that we mistakenly believe is "somewhere out there" which prevents us from dieting the way we must in order to accomplish our goal of losing body fat.

There are several ways to burn more calories than you eat. You can add more cardiovascular work to your training regimen, simply eat less food throughout the day, or even do a combination of more cardiovascular training and eating less food.

Can I build muscle and lose fat at the same time?

One question I am continually asked is, "Is it possible to lose body fat and gain muscle at the same time?" My answer is an emphatic yes!

First of all, to build muscle, you must constantly overload the muscles in the gym. Heavy training is of utmost importance. Even when you are on a calorie-deprived diet to lose body fat, you must be mentally tough and continue to train heavily to preserve and even build muscle mass. And, as I've discussed several times already, back up heavy training by eating high-quality protein on a consistent basis.

To lose body fat and still gain muscle, you must really watch your diet closely. Keep your daily caloric intake below your maintenance level. When you reduce your calories, be sure to keep your diet high in quality protein. **Most of your calories should come from your protein consumption.** Of course, watch your fat intake.

> The Doctor Says:
> Building muscle and losing bodyfat at the same time is a process that is a natural defense mechanism for the body. Don't let others mislead you when they say it can't be done, they just don't know all the facts.

Here is how I suggest you manipulate your carbohydrate consumption: For a couple of days, eat only vegetables for carbohydrates then go back to grains like rice, potatoes, and pasta for a couple of days. Rotate in this manner and see how quickly you start melting the fat. Because carbohydrates give you energy, this may become difficult at times. Nevertheless, it is a very effective strategy.

Getting shredded and keeping mass

I believe getting ripped is a matter of having a little bit of knowledge, but most important, having a lot of "heart". It takes a lot of discipline to stay on your diet for a longer time than others who have faster metabolisms or who use chemicals to assist them.

You have to go hungry sometimes while continuing to train hard and heavy so you can retain as much muscle as possible. I believe many more drug-free bodybuilders could be in better condition. **It is a matter of whether or not they are willing to do the hard work and go through the sacrifice that's required.**

Fat-burning mode: learn to love it

Over the years, I've learned to become acute to my body's signals that let me know if I'm on the right track to gradually lose fat. I can tell when I am turning my body into a "fat-burning machine" or in other words, when I feel as though my body is running at an optimal fat-burning mode. What does that feel like? Well, for starters, I have that "hungry-but-not-hungry feeling" most of the time. My stomach never feels full, even immediately after eating a meal. The most I ever feel is satisfied. My body temperature is much hotter throughout the day and I am sweating more profusely during my cardiovascular sessions.

Many bodybuilders get "freaked out" when they see what their body looks like when it's in fat-burning mode. They fear that they are getting small and losing muscle. Visually, my body does appear to be smaller and my clothes fit more loosely. My muscle-bellies are much flatter than when I'm eating more food. It's not that I'm losing muscle; it's just that my muscles are not filled with as much glycogen, therefore look like deflated balloons. This is a necessary evil; at least for a period of time.

I have learned over the years to associate positive emotions to these kinesthetic-external and visual feelings during the dieting process, not fear. These are sure-fire indicators that I am well on my way to being in the shape I want and the look that I am going for.

Top 7 Fitness Success Formulas

If there's one thing we've learned by now, it's that the drastic, cut out all (carbs, fat, protein, sugar, dairy, eggs, calories heck - why not everything?) Diets are not the answer to the energy and physique you want. Sure, you're going to drop some pounds pretty fast, but they're unlikely to stay away very long.

Now, there are two schools of thought when it comes to making major changes in your life. Some experts agree that making small changes in your diet and activity level will add up to a slow and steady weight loss. And the simpler they are, the more likely you'll stick with them for the rest of your life.

These experts reason that if you make a really dramatic change, you'll be so overwhelmed that you'll just go back to what you were doing before. Sounds good, doesn't it? It's like they're saying, "You can still make changes, but you don't have to get out of your comfort zone to do it."

Here's the deal: while we generally know what to do and how to do it, there needs to be a catalyst of some sort to ignite the change process. But doing something you're used to doing will keep getting you the results you've been getting.

Massive action, man. Get out of that comfort zone. DO IT.

Be confident and take BIG steps to change. Create momentum for yourself so that you become unstoppable. Having a leaner, energized, body with confidence and determination is important to you, SO GO GET IT. Let others know what you're doing to give yourself more leverage to keep at it.

The math is simple. To lose a pound of fat you need to burn 3500 more calories than you take in. So if you burn 200 calories from working out and shave 300 calories from what you normally eat in a day, you'll lose that pound of fat.

If you want to lose 1.5 pounds of fat, bump up the intensity of your exercise. I don't recommend cutting your calories drastically, since you need to feed your body nourishing food for it to perform at its best, protect muscle, have energy, and mental performance.

So if you burn an extra 250 calories on top of the 200 you're already burning (and it's easy to do), you can lose the 1.5 pounds of fat. A 30-minute strength training workout can incinerate 200-500 calories. Compliment it with aerobics, and you're on your way to melting off 12 pounds of ugly fat in about two months.

Take a look at this list of seven mini-recipes for your health and fitness success. DO THEM. If they're not working for you, re-word them so that they do. The goal is to simplify the success process.

1. Listen to your body

Are you truly hungry when you eat, or do you end to snack out of habit without paying attention to your appetite? If you're eating when you're not hungry, those are usually extra calories that your body doesn't need.

So, before you reach for a snack, ask yourself if you're physically hungry. Sometimes hunger is a sign of thirst, so try drinking a big glass of water and see if your appetite subsides. If you are physically hungry, eat a nutritious, balanced snack.

FORMULAS:
STOP + ASK = SAVE CALORIES
STOP/ASK + DRINK WATER = CONTROL APPETITE

2. Control your portions

Many of us tend to eat more serving of low-fat or fat-free foods like bread, bagels, cereals, and desserts than we realize. We hear too much about cutting out the fat, but not enough of "control your portions."

Check the labels to compare its portion size to what you're really eating. You may be in for an eye-opener. A half-cup of pasta is about 200 calories, so a plateful of pasta could end up being some 600 calories, NOT including sauce, bread, and meat or protein source. Wow. Now you're talking a potential 1000 calorie dinner.

Then there's the "dining out challenge." Look, you don't HAVE to eat what they've served you. Eat maybe a third of what's on your plate, then bring the rest home. That way you'll still feel satisfied.

You also don't have to measure your portions. Use the palm of your hand as a measuring device. The "eyeball method," I call it. For veggies, fill 2-3 palmsful for a serving; fruits, 1 palmful; protein, 1 palmful; and fat, the round line around your thumb area (about 1-2 tsp.)

FORMULAS:
CHECK LABEL + STICK WITH THAT SERVING SIZE = SAVE CALORIES
DINE OUT + CUT PORTIONS BY 1/3 = CUT CALORIES
EYEBALL METHOD + BALANCE MEALS = MORE NUTRITION WITH LESS CALORIES

3. Slow down!

If you're a fast eater, try these two tips for helping you eat less and still feel satisfied:

1. At the beginning of your meal, eat something you can't consume quickly, like hot soup or spicy salsa. If you're forced to slow down, you'll give your body a chance to feel satisfied before you overeat.

2. Put your fork or spoon down in between bites, and keep the TV or radio off. It takes about 20 minutes for you to feel full, so take time to enjoy your food instead of scarfing it down.

FORMULAS:
"SPEED BUMP" FOOD + SLOW DOWN = SATISFACTION WITHOUT OVEREATING
PUT FORK/SPOON DOWN + QUIET SETTING = ENJOY FOOD & FEEL SATISFIED

4. Substitute smarter

Look at foods you regularly eat and try to cut calories that you won't miss. For instance, if you always eat a scrambled egg with breakfast, scramble two egg whites. Or substitute mustard for mayonnaise on your sandwich. Try the new Pam cooking sprays that are butter, olive, or garlic flavored on your cooked veggies instead of butter.

FORMULA:
FOOD + SUBSTITUTE = CUT CALORIES WITHOUT CUTTING FLAVOR

5. What are you drinking?

If you regularly down lattes, cafe mochas, or sweetened beverages, you're drinking more calories than you realize. Research has shown that people don't think of beverages as food. If you have a couple of glasses of orange juice for breakfast, that's at least 300 calories right there.

Cutting back on coffee and tea can have a marked improvement on your weight if you normally add cream and sugar. Little things make a huge difference.

FORMULAS:
NORMAL BEVERAGE + DRINK STRAIGHT = SAVE CALORIES
ATTITUDE ABOUT DRINK + SUBSTITUTE OR ELIMINATE = CUT CALORIES

6. Get your butt in gear

Of course you knew I was going to mention exercise at some point in this article. You just can't overlook the calorie-burning benefits of exercise. Now exercise is not just about aerobics and lifting weights. You can burn a good amount of calories by doing housework or yard work with some vigor. Remember, LITTLE THINGS… Also remember, LIFE IS EXERCISE. So shoot for 30 minutes each day.

FORMULA:
EXERCISE + DAILY = SERIOUS CALORIE BURNING

7. Join your kids

Just because you're running around with your kids with their activities doesn't mean you can't be active yourself. Going to your kid's soccer game? Walk around the field while you're watching.

Get them involved with physical fitness. If your kids are old enough, make it a family-thing to go for a walk together, or a bike ride. If you're watching TV, make it a game and see how many push ups each of you can do during commercials (or crunches) before the show comes back on.

FORMULA:
FAMILY + ACTIVITY = EXTRA CALORIE BURNING AND FIT FAMILY
KIDS' ACTIVITIES + ACTIVE WATCHING ACTIVITY = NO EXCUSE FOR "NO TIME"

8. Build muscle!

If you want to achieve lasting weight loss, be SURE to include strength training into your fitness routine. You know the story: lean muscle increases your metabolism, allowing you to burn more calories even at rest; you're stronger, so you fatigue less often and not as quickly; you melt off fat faster, so you can sculpt a great looking body.

FORMULAS:
STRENGTH TRAINING + METABOLISM = LASTING WEIGHT LOSS
STRENGTH TRAINING + PROPER NUTRITION = HIGH METABOLISM
STRENGTH TRAINING + AEROBIC CONDITIONING = ENERGY, VITALITY, BODY YOU WANT

<u>The dangers of excess body fat</u>

Most people's primary motivation for weight management is to improve their appearance. Equally important, however, are the many other benefits of proper nutrition and regular exercise.

Weight management through reduction of excess body fat plays a vital role in maintaining good health and fighting disease. In fact, medical evidence shows that obesity poses a major threat to health and longevity. The most common definition of obesity is more than 25 percent body fat for men and more than 32 percent for women. **An estimated one in three Americans has some excess body fat; an estimated 20 percent are obese.** Excess body fat is linked to major physical threats like heart disease, cancer, and diabetes.

For example, if you're obese, it takes more energy for you to breathe because your heart has to work harder to pump blood to the lungs and to the excess fat throughout the body. This increased workload can cause your heart to become enlarged and can result in high blood pressure and life-threatening erratic heartbeats.

Obese people also tend to have high cholesterol levels, making them more prone to arteriosclerosis, a narrowing of the arteries by deposits of plaque. This becomes life threatening when blood vessels become so narrow or blocked that vital organs like the brain, heart or kidneys are deprived of blood. Additionally, the narrowing of the blood vessels forces the heart to pump harder, and blood pressure rises. High blood pressure itself poses several health risks, including heart attack, kidney failure, and stroke. About 25 percent of all heart and blood vessel problems are associated with obesity.

Clinical studies have found a relationship between excess body fat and the incidence of cancer. By itself, body fat is thought to be a storage place for carcinogens (cancer-causing chemicals) in both men and women. In women, excess body fat has been linked to a higher rate of breast and uterine cancer; in men, the threat comes from colon and prostate cancer.

There is also a delicate balance between blood sugar, body fat, and the hormone insulin. Excess blood sugar is stored in the liver and other vital organs; when the organs are "full," the excess blood sugar is converted to fat. As fat cells themselves become full, they tend to take in less blood sugar. In some obese people, the pancreas produces more and more insulin, which the body can't use, to regulate blood sugar levels, and the whole system becomes overwhelmed. This poor regulation of blood sugar and insulin results in diabetes, a disease with long-term consequences, including heart disease, kidney failure, blindness, amputation, and death. Excess body fat is also linked to gall bladder disease, gastro-intestinal disease, sexual dysfunction, osteoarthritis, and stroke.

Reducing body fat reduces disease risk

The good news is that reducing body fat reduces the risk of disease. At the University of Pittsburgh, researchers studied 159 people as they followed a weight management program. The subjects were under age 45 and 30-70 pounds overweight. Those subjects who were able to shed just 10-15 percent of their weight and keep it off during the 18-month study showed significant improvement in HDL cholesterol and triglyceride levels, waist-to-hip ratio, and blood pressure. In fact, according to the New England Journal of Medicine, body fat reduction is a more powerful modulator of cardiac structure than drug therapy.

For people with a family history of heart disease, an active lifestyle can slow or stop the process for all but those with serious genetic disorders. Studies by Dr. Dean Ornish, have shown that a comprehensive intervention program that includes regular physical activity, a low-fat diet and a stress reduction program can even reverse the heart disease process.

Evidence also shows that an active lifestyle and its help in reducing body fat is associated with a reduced risk for some types of cancers: prostate for men, breast and uterine cancers for women. Just a few more reasons to get into weightlifting!

In addition, regular physical activity and a low-fat diet are successful in treating non-insulin dependent diabetes (NIDDM); for some patients, it has reduced or eliminated the need for insulin substitutes. In general, regularly active adults have 42 percent lower risk of developing NIDDM.

Gaining fat happens to us naturally

The average American gains at least one pound a year after age 25. Think about it. If you're like most Americans, by the time you're 50, you're likely to gain 25 pounds of fat, or more. In addition, your metabolism is also slowing down, causing your body to work less efficiently at burning the fat it has. At the same time, if you don't exercise regularly, you lose a pound of muscle each year. Consequently, people are not only increasing their body fat stores, increasing their risk of disease, but they're also losing muscle, increasing the risk of injury, decreasing activity performance, and further slowing down metabolism.

Very few Americans exercise in any significant way. The President's Council on Physical Fitness and Sports estimates that only one in five Americans exercises for the healthy minimum of 20 minutes, three or more days a week. In fact, the average American gets less than 50 minutes of exercise per week. Even worse, two out of five Americans are completely sedentary.

Healthy eating and fitness are the best defenses against being fat

But there is hope. Moderate weight loss, of fat, not muscle, and a healthy and active lifestyle, not dieting; have been found to lower health risks and medical problems in 90 percent of overweight patients. Improving their heart function, blood pressure, glucose tolerance, sleep disorders, and cholesterol levels, as well as lowering their requirements for medication, lowering the incidence and duration of hospitalization, and reducing postoperative complications. **Fit people are also eight times less likely to die from heart disease.**

So, are you willing to be patient and make the changes in your life that will lead to a healthier, happier you? Once you have made the decision to go forward and accept change, the hard part is over. Sure, there is plenty of work to be done, but it really doesn't matter how long this new process takes. If you allow changes to take place over the course of a year, your body will adjust comfortably, and you will be more likely to maintain the healthy lifestyle permanently.

When you begin achieving improvements in energy and physical and psychological performance, the fun and excitement you experience will make the change well worth the effort. Action creates motivation! Good luck: I hope you enjoy all the wonderful benefits of a safe and effective weight management program.

Turning fat into muscle myth

Many health and fitness magazines alike splash the wonderful promise of turning fat into muscle on their covers once in a while. **You simply cannot transform fat tissue into muscle. Muscles mass and fat are two different animals:** Muscle is active tissue that burns calories around the clock even as you sleep, kind of like an engine running in neutral. When you move around, you burn more calories, just like a car will consume more gas the faster you go.

Fat, on the other hand, is just storage of excess energy. It does nothing but sit there with its sole goal in life to be a spare tire around your waist until you put in the effort to burn it off. Bodyfat is not particularly useful except as padding against bumps, as insulation to preserve warmth, and as a convenient surface where you can balance a can of beer while watching the game, as frequently demonstrated by my potbellied neighbor. You need some bodyfat to stay healthy of course, but unless you're walking around with razor-sharp abs and sunken-in, fat-depleted cheeks year-round, you probably have nothing to fear.

Having recognized the difference between the two, let's get down to business: Getting rid of the fat and grow the muscles. It can be difficult to achieve both goals at the same time. The reason for this is that in order to maintain an environment in your body that facilitates fat burn, you must deplete yourself of calories. Growth requires extra calories, much like you'd need extra building material to add a room to your house. In addition, **insulin, which is a key component of growing muscle, is the anti-Christ of fat burn and is released whenever you eat carbohydrates.** How much and how fast depends entirely on the type of carbs, however.

I recommend beginning by trying to pack on the muscle. That means you'll have to eat extra calories, including the extra carbs, and live with the fact that you'll probably gain a few pounds of lard in the process. There's no need to worry about this as long as you keep the increase in bodyfat under control and avoid ballooning like the Pillsbury Doughboy. **Train heavy; eat lots of healthy bodybuilding food (pasta, rice, chicken, lean beef, tuna, oatmeal etc.) but no junk food, candy or alcohol.**

When you've packed on perhaps 5 or 10 pounds of muscle (or whatever your goal was,) switch gears and start the diet. As always, you'll have to keep a daily log of what you eat and carefully adjust your eating patterns so that you eat an average of 500 calories less than you burn each day. Here's where you reap the benefit of having gained the muscle beforehand: Remember the analogy of your muscles being like an engine running in neutral? Muscle burn calories 24/7, and the more mass you have, the more calories are burned without you even having to lift a finger. This in turn translates to a more lenient diet. In other words, if your added muscle mass boosts your natural metabolism by, say 200 calories per day, **that's 200 calories more you can eat and STILL lose bodyfat!** In other words, you'll look better, get to eat more, and will still lose fat at the same rate.

The Doctor Says:
During your fat loss training / diet regimen you need to keep up your protein intake. This will help spare the amino acids in your muscles from being consumed and protein foods make you feel fuller so you can keep your total calories low.

As you diet, you want to keep the protein intake up. Also make sure to keep hitting the weights as you did before; it's your best insurance policy against losing your hard earned muscle mass. The goal at this point is to slowly but surely shave off the fat without sacrificing mass, so take it easy. No sudden changes in eating habits will improve your situation; only worsen it. After a few months you should have lost at least 10-15 lbs of fat, and if you played your cards right, you should have kept most of the gains you made prior to the diet. By taking a little more time and splitting up your two goals, you achieved what you wanted.

Cardiovascular exercise principles and guidelines

One of the most common myths out there in the gyms seem to be that cardiovascular training equals loss of muscle mass. Period. End of story. And it just won't go away. That is also why you seldom see the hardcore gym rats leave the power rack to join the ladies by the Stairmasters. Who in turn believe in the myth of females suddenly gaining a hundred pounds of muscle by even smelling a barbell.

Needless to say, both categories of trainers are in fact robbing themselves of optimal results. The women would get firmer, stronger and leaner if they'd throw in 2-3 sessions of weight training. And the men would experience several advantages if they'd pick up cardiovascular training.

Oxygen

With every breath you take, you breathe in oxygen, which is absorbed by the blood in your lungs. I guess most of you remember all that stuff from your biology classes so I won't go into depth in it, and besides it doesn't really matter in your daily life. What does matter, however, are two things:

1. Your physical capability is closely connected to your oxygen intake.

2. You can improve it.

"Sure," someone says, "If I were a marathon-runner I'd care, but I'm a bodybuilder. And I've done my homework; bodybuilding is anaerobic work, not aerobic! Why should I give a crap?"

You're right about the anaerobic part, but you need oxygen, even if you make a minimum amount of reps, say 4 heavy reps of deadlifts, are you trying to tell me you're not the least out of breath afterwards? Right, you come up with an oxygen deficit. And here's news for you, the less oxygen available, and the more lactic buildup you get. Besides, do you *always* do extreme low-rep training? Improving the cardiovascular capacity is a good way of avoiding those dancing black spots in your vision at the end of a high-rep set. And in case your training partner isn't buying any of this, just tell him to do 20 reps of squatting with a plastic bag over his head and I'm sure he'll see the importance of oxygen, even in anaerobic training.

Heart

This must be one of the oldest facts in popular medicine, so I'll make it really simple: Regular cardiovascular exercise strengthens your heart and makes you live longer. It also lowers your resting heart rate and lowers your blood pressure. Questions?

Fat loss

With this kind of exercise, you have a much better chance of getting rid of the love handles as opposed to if you'd rely solely on weight training. As numerous tests have shown, it's a simple, sane combination of both that yields the best results. So what happens? Well, for one thing, for fat burn to take place you need oxygen available. It needs it. **No oxygen = carbs used for fuel.** And like I said before, that only results in lactic acid used for fuel and is an extremely inefficient way to get energy. ***More oxygen = better fat burn.***

Then there's details such as improved amount of mitochondria (the unit of the cell that burns fat), decreased levels of fat in the bloodstream, increased amount of fine capillaries, better blood pressure and so on.

Killing the myth

So, all this is fine and dandy. But what about the muscle mass? Don't worry, it ain't going anywhere! Two important things though: You must eat. If you do not eat properly, the body inevitably has to use stored energy. Sure, some fat might get burned but your muscle is more of a prime target as starvation = fat burn shutdown. And as muscle is "active", i.e. burns energy 24 hours a day, the best thing for the body to do, it thinks, is to shed excessive muscle, thus saving fat and reduce future energy loss. It's self-preservation, according to our ancestors.

The second thing to think about is not to overdo it. If you exercise for 4 hours straight you're in the danger zone. Experts talk about 60 minutes as the max for a weight training session to last, as after that your carb storage in your body is out and your hormone balance starts to really work against you. I haven't read any studies on muscle mass / long term cardiovascular training, but take a good look at a marathon runner make an educated guess. ***However, I'd like to underline this: if you do watch out for these two obvious potholes, you have nothing but gains to expect from this!***

Mental aspects

No need to dwell on the physiological part, it's good for you, plain and simple. But it's also good to do something else than go to the same gym, lifting the same weights, day in and day out. Go mountain biking in the weekends! Play basketball! Go swim! What you do is really not that important, as long as you do something out of the gym for a change! And guess what? By breaking out of the rut, perhaps even going hiking in the mountains for a week can actually prove extremely productive for your bodybuilding goals! Not only do you let your muscles rest, you also get overall, moderate body stimulation in a way they're not used to! Result: You can come back and attack the weights like a new person. Remember, your biggest enemies are boredom and routine!

Now that we know that cardiovascular training, or plain "cardio", isn't the antagonist of muscle as it's rumored to be, it's time to get down to action! Let's be honest for a second. It's the gym that's priority #1; cardio is more of a necessary evil, *unless you make it fun!*

I can play basketball for hours. Not only am I keeping my pulse up for much longer, I'm also having a ball, which motivates me to come back and do it again. For a guy like me, the difference would be approx. 1000 cal / hour (running) vs. 800 cal / hour (basketball). But as I'd be able to play basketball for, say 5 hours a week (easily) I'd only be able to get 2 hours of running, 2.5 hours if I'm pushing it. And simple math tells us that 5 x 800 sums up to more than 2000 or 2500 cal. Which cardio program do you think will still have me as a follower a month later? Bottom line: Forget those fancy calories-per-hour charts! The three criteria for your cardio training schedule should be:

1. You think its fun.

2. It gets the heart rate up (65% of max for fat burn, 80% for endurance)

3. It doesn't contradict your bodybuilding goals.

Point 1 is easy, while points 2 and 3 might need some clarification. Your target heart rate depends on the particular goal you have with your cardio. Is the cardio a part of a fat-loss program? In that case, go easy and make sure not to get your heart rate up too much! If you do, you run a risk of losing too much muscle mass.

However, if you're bulking up or just want to remain fit, you want to keep the heart in top shape and possibly improving the overall capacity. Then you should aim for higher heart rates, where 80% of max is a good rule of thumb. **The max is decided by your age, as in: 220 - age = approximate max pulse.** A 30-year old person would be: 220 - 30 = 190 max.

Point 3 is quite logical. Example: Your lats are skinny, and you feel like adding some muscle onto them. Then rowing might not be a good choice for cardio, as you run a fair risk of overtraining your back, while dancing or power walking allows your back to rest while still getting your cardio done. It's pretty simple; don't choose a cardio activity that uses the same muscles you're trying to grow the most.

Beware

Before you get all Gung-Ho about it and start out with high set goals, make an honest evaluation of your own shape. What's my history? Is my schedule realistic? Can I stick to this schedule for more than two weeks? And if you have any heart or respiratory problems, make sure to consult a physician before taking on a serious program. And do I even have to mention it? If you have asthma, you don't do anything without proper medication available! For the rest of you: Just listen to your body, and you're on the highway to excellence!

For maximum effectiveness and safety, cardiovascular exercise has specific instructions on the frequency, duration, and intensity. These are the three important components of cardiovascular exercise that you really need to understand and implement in your program. In addition, your cardiovascular program should include a warm-up, a cool-down, and stretching of the primary muscles used in the exercise.

Warming up and stretching

One very common mistake is stretching before muscles are warmed-up. It is important to stretch after your muscles are warm, after blood has circulated through them. **Never stretch a cold muscle. First warm up.** A warm-up should be done for at least 3-7 minutes at a low intensity. Usually, the warm-up is done by doing the same activity as the cardiovascular workout but at an intensity of 50-60% of maximum heart rate. After you've warmed-up for 3-7 minutes at a relatively low intensity, your muscles should be warm. To prevent injury and to improve your performance, you should stretch the primary muscles used in the warm up before proceeding to the cardiovascular exercise.

Cooling down

The cool down is similar to the warm-up in that it should last 3-7 minutes and be done at a low intensity (50-60% of max HR). After you have completed your cardiovascular exercise and cooled-down properly, it is now important that you stretch the primary muscles that were used. **Warming-up, stretching, and cooling-down** are very important to every exercise session. They not only help your performance levels and produce better results; they **also drastically decrease your risk of injury.**

Frequency of exercise

The first component of cardiovascular exercise is frequency of the exercise, which refers to the number of exercise sessions per week. To improve both cardiovascular fitness and to decrease body fat or maintain body fat at optimum levels, **you should exercise cardiovascularly, at least three days a week.** The American College of Sports Medicine recommends three to five days a week for most cardiovascular programs.

> The Doctor Says:
> My cardio part of the workout lasts for 20-30 minutes and I do it 3-4 days a week. Do this consistently and this is all it takes to lose body fat and keep your heart healthy.

Those of you who are very out of shape and/or who are overweight and doing weight-bearing cardiovascular exercise such as an aerobics class or jogging, might want to have at least 36 to 48 hours of rest between workouts to prevent an injury and to promote adequate bone and joint stress recovery.

Duration of exercise

The second component of cardiovascular exercise is the duration, which refers to the time you've spent exercising. The cardiovascular session, not including the warm-up and cool-down, should vary from 20-40 minutes to gain significant cardio respiratory and fat burning-benefits. Each time you do your cardiovascular exercise; **try to do at least 20 minutes or more.** Of course, the longer you go, the more calories and fat you'll burn and the better you'll condition your cardiovascular system. All beginners, especially those who are out of shape, should take a very conservative approach and train at relatively low intensities (50-70% max HR) for 10-20 minutes. As you get in better shape, you can gradually increase the duration of time you exercise.

It is important that you gradually increase the duration before you increase the intensity. That is, when beginning a walking program for example, be more concerned with increasing the number of minutes of the exercise session before you increase the intensity, by increasing your speed or by walking hilly terrain.

Remember that cardiovascular exercise should be done a minimum of three times a week and a minimum of 20 minutes per session. Once your muscles are warm and after the cardiovascular exercise, you should stretch those muscles used in the exercise. For example, after bicycling, stretch your quadriceps, hamstrings, calves, hips, and low back. After doing the rowing machine, stretch your legs, back, biceps, and shoulders. Good luck and enjoy all the wonderful benefits of cardiovascular exercise.

There are several ways to monitor the exercise intensity. The best way to test the intensity is to take your heart rate during the exercise, within the first 5 minutes of your cardiovascular exercise session and again just before the cool-down.

There are two ways in which you can check your heart rate during exercise. The most accurate one is to purchase a heart-rate monitor that you strap around your chest. It will give you feedback on a digital watch that tells you exactly what your heart rate is at a specific time in the exercise session. The other way to obtain your heart rate is by palpating (feeling) the carotid artery, the temporal artery, or the radial artery. The easiest site is either the carotid or the radial artery. The carotid artery may be felt by gently placing your index finger on your neck, between the middle of your collarbone and jaw line. Placing your index and middle finger on the underside and thumb-side of your wrist does palpating the radial artery.

When you're taking your heart rate you measure it in beats per minute. **For convenience, many people take their pulse for 6 seconds and multiply that number by 10, or simply add a 0 behind the number just obtained.** So, if in 6 seconds you counted 12 beats, which would mean your heart rate was 120 beats per minute (bpm). Although counting for 6 seconds is most convenient, keep in mind that the longer the time interval used, the more accurate the results will be. For example, counting your heart rate for 30 seconds and then multiplying that number by 2 will give a slightly more accurate reading than counting your heart rate for 15 seconds and multiplying by 4, or 10 seconds and multiplying by 6. Whatever time interval you use, be consistent.

Heart zone training gets the most out of cardio work

How do you know if you are training too intensely or not intensely enough for what you want to achieve? This is where Heart Zone Training comes in. This is different for everyone. To use Heart Zone Training you must first determine your maximum heart rate.

You can determine your max HR one of two ways. One way is to use the age predicted max HR formula, whereby you subtract your age from 220. So, if you were 40 years old, your predicted max HR would be 180 bpm. The other method, which is much more accurate and more individualized, is actually having a medical or fitness professional administer a max HR test for you, which is usually done on a stationery bicycle or treadmill for several minutes and requires very hard work. Thus, only those cleared by a physician should do this test. I do not explain how to administer this test because only trained professionals should do so.

Once you have determined your max HR, you will need to decide what zone you want to train at. There are five different training zones separated by 10% increments, each having different characteristics and benefits.

Healthy heart zone

The first zone is called the Healthy Heart Zone. **This is 50-60% of your max HR.** This is the easiest and most comfortable zone within which to train and is the one that is best for people who are just starting an exercise program or have low functional capacity. Those of you who are walkers most likely train at this zone. Although this zone has been criticized for not burning enough total calories, and for not being intense enough to get great cardio respiratory benefits, **it has been shown to help decrease body fat, blood pressure and cholesterol.** It also decreases the risk of degenerative diseases and has a low risk of injury. **In this zone, 10% of carbohydrates are "burned" (used as energy), 5% of protein is burned and a whopping 85% of fat is burned.**

Fitness zone

The next zone is the Fitness Zone, **which is 60-70% of your max HR. Once again, 85% of your calories burned in this zone are fats, 5% are proteins and 10% are carbohydrates.** Studies have shown that in this zone you can condition your fat mobilization (getting fat out of your cells) while conditioning your fat transportation (getting fat to the muscles). Thus, in this zone, you are training your fat cells to increase the rate of fat release and training your muscles to burn fat. Therefore, the benefits of this zone are not only the same as the healthy heart zone training at 50-60% but you are now slightly increasing the total number of calories burned and provide a little more cardio respiratory benefits. You burn more total calories at this zone simply because it is more intense.

Aerobic zone

The third zone, the Aerobic Zone, requires that you **train at 70-80% of your max HR.** This is the preferred zone if you are training for an endurance event. In this zone, your functional capacity will greatly improve and you can expect to increase the number and size of blood vessels, increase vital capacity and respiratory rate and achieve increases in pulmonary ventilation, as well as increases in arterial venous oxygen. Moreover, stroke volume (amount of blood pumped per heart beat) will increase, and your resting heart rate will decrease.

What does all this mean? It means that your cardiovascular and respiratory system will improve and you will increase the size and strength of your heart. **In this zone, 50% of calories burned are from carbohydrates, 50% are from fat and less than 1% is from protein.** And, because there is an increase in intensity, there is also an increase in the total number of calories burned.

Anaerobic zone

The next training zone is called the Threshold or Anaerobic zone, which is 80-90% of your max HR. Benefits include an improved VO2 maximum, the highest amount of oxygen one can consume during exercise. And thus an improved cardio respiratory system, and a higher lactate tolerance ability, which means your endurance, will improve and you'll be able to fight fatigue better. Since the intensity is high, more calories will be burned than within the other three zones. Although more calories are burned in this zone, **85% of the calories burned are from carbohydrates, 15% from fat and less than 1% is from protein.**

Red-line zone

The last training zone is called **the Redline Zone, which is 90-100% of your max HR.** Remember, training at 100% is your maximum heart rate; your heart rate will not get any higher. This zone burns the highest total number of calories and the lowest percentage of fat calories. **Ninety percent of the calories burned here are carbohydrates, only 10% are fats and again less than one percent is protein.** This zone is so intense that very few people can actually stay in this zone for the minimum 20 minutes, or even five minutes. You should only train in this zone if you are in very good shape and have been cleared by a physician to do so. Usually, people use this zone for interval training. For example, one might do three minutes in the Aerobic Zone and then one minute in this Redline Zone and then back to the Aerobic Zone.

Your greatest challenge, however, is not learning new cardiovascular exercises or the proper technique. It's not learning the heart rate zone to train at for your goals and interests or how to monitor the intensity. Nor is it deciding when to try new cardiovascular exercises. The greatest challenge facing you at this moment is deciding whether you are willing to take action and make time for yourself and make cardiovascular exercise a priority.

When you begin achieving great results, the excitement and fun you experience will make the change well worth the effort. Action creates motivation! Good luck: I hope you enjoy all the wonderful benefits of an effective cardiovascular exercise program.

Getting in great shape by spending only twenty minutes a day, three days a week sounds great. There are plenty of "guru's" out there claiming that "Eight minutes a day on the XYZ machine is all it takes" or "Just twenty minutes a day is the solution," but when things sound too good to be true, they usually are.

If your goal is better health and a decent level of cardiovascular fitness, then three days of cardio a week for 20 minutes is all you need. However, if your goal is to lose a lot of body fat as quickly as possible, then you're probably going to need a lot more than 20 minutes.

If you're one of the few people who are genetically blessed with a fast metabolism and the ability to burn fat easily, then three days a week for twenty minutes will work for you. In fact, I know a few people with hyperactive metabolisms that stay ripped all year round without doing any cardio at all! Not many people are that fortunate.

I've seen very few people who can lose fat quickly from just three days a week of cardio. On the other hand, I have never seen anyone do six days a week of cardio for 45 minutes and not lose a lot of body fat. Provided of course, that they were on a good diet.

It's true that moderate to high intensity cardio such as interval training is more effective than low intensity cardio: The higher the intensity, the more calories you burn. The problem is that you can only burn so many calories in 20 minutes. The more calories you burn in a one-week period, the more fat you'll lose. If you do a high intensity interval workout 3 times a week for 20 minutes on a Stairmaster or bike at a high intensity, you might burn about 400 calories. That's a lot of calories for a twenty-minute workout. But it only adds up to 1200 total calories burned in one week. If you doubled your time to 40 minutes and you did six days per week at a moderate intensity, you would burn about 600 calories per workout. Do that 6 times per week and that's a total of 3600 calories in a week; three times as much as the high intensity interval workout! Combine the cardio with a 500-calorie per day deficit and that's another 3500 calories for a total deficit of 7100 calories per week. **There are 3500 calories in a pound of fat,** so that's two pounds of fat you'd lose in one week!

What I would suggest is that you approach your cardio training in cycles depending on what your goals are. If you just want to maintain your current level of body fat and stay healthy, I'd recommend 20-30 minutes of aerobic activity 3 - 4 times per week. If your goal is maximum fat loss, then I'd recommend 30-60 minutes 5-7 days per week. Once you reach your desired percentage of bodyfat, then you could drop down to just 3 - 4 days a week for 20 minutes to maintain your low body fat level.

I agree that low intensity cardio is not the best way to lose fat. You should always keep your intensity moderate to high, provided that you can maintain it for the desired duration. If you reach 45-60 minutes six times per week and you're still not losing fat, then the problem is definitely your diet, not your workout program.

The bottom line is that you should do as much or as little cardio as it takes for you to reach your goal. You can only determine how much that is by getting started and then learning through trial and error. If you can lose fat from just three 20 minute workouts a week- that's GREAT! Don't do more if you don't have to. However, if you've been doing

20 minute workouts three times per week and nothing is happening, then you need to increase your duration and/or frequency until the fat starts coming off.

Calories burned in selected activities

Activity	Calories burned per hour
Bicycling, 6 mph	240
Bicycling, 12 mph	410
Cross-country skiing	700
Jogging, 5½ mph	740
Jogging, 7 mph	920
Jumping rope	50
Running in place	650
Running, 10 mph	1280
Swimming, 25 yds./min.	275
Swimming, 50 yds./min.	500
Tennis, singles	400
Walking, 2 mph	240
Walking, 3 mph	320
Walking, 4½ mph	440

Target heart rates by age

Age	Target heart rate zone
20 years	100 - 150 beats per minute
25 years	98 - 146 beats per minute
30 years	95 - 142 beats per minute
35 years	93 - 138 beats per minute
40 years	90 - 135 beats per minute
45 years	88 - 131 beats per minute
50 years	85 - 127 beats per minute
55 years	83 - 123 beats per minute
60 years	80 - 120 beats per minute
65 years	78 - 116 beats per minute
70 years	75 - 113 beats per minute

<u>Best time of day for cardio</u>

WARNING: What you are about to read is the answer to the most common question people have about their cardio/aerobic workout. What you are about to read is all 100% true! What you are about to read is the answer to the question that personal trainers and fitness magazines will make you pay for. Enjoy.

This is another time where what I am writing is inspired by questions people have mailed to me. So, be sure to keep those questions coming so I have more material to write about.

Now, on to the question. When is the best time of day to do cardio, and why? Well, I bet most people do cardio "whenever they get a chance." Sometimes during the middle of the day, sometimes before bed, sometimes directly after your weightlifting workout, sometimes directly before the weightlifting workout and sometimes first thing in the morning. The truth is, all of those times will get results. It doesn't matter what time of day you do your cardio workout, you will be burning calories every time. But, the real question is, which of those times is the most effective? And the answer is**… first thing in the morning!**

Doing cardio first thing in the morning, on an empty stomach, before you eat anything, is by far, the most effective. Whether you run, jog, walk, swim, jump rope, take an aerobics class, ride a bike, etc., doing it first thing in the morning is the best time to do it for maximum fat loss. Why? It's simple. When you do your cardio workout, you are burning calories. Lets say you wake up, eat breakfast, eat lunch later in the day, and then a few hours after lunch, you do your cardio. All you will be doing during that cardio session is burning the calories and carbs of the food you just ate. When you do cardio first thing in the morning, you haven't eaten anything for the last 8 or so hours because you were sleeping. So, **when your body sees that there are no carbs to burn, it goes directly to stored bodyfat.** And stored bodyfat is the fat that is on your body, which is the fat that you want to lose!

Understand how it works? When you do your cardio sometime during the day other then first thing in the morning, you spend most of that time burning off carbs that you already ate that day. When you do it first thing in the morning, there are no carbs to burn, so all your body can burn is body fat!

Doctor's Prescription:
Do your cardio work first thing in the morning for the synergistic benefit of cardiovascular exercise and fat loss. Do cardio at any other time of day for the cardiovascular exercise benefit only.

Some people have e-mailed me asking what type of cardio I do and I tell them I jog on my treadmill first thing in the morning. Even though I do all of my weightlifting at a gym, I do my cardio in my house on my own treadmill so I can do it first thing in the morning without having to take a shower, get dressed and do whatever else I'd do if I went to the gym to do cardio.

Monitoring your fat loss progress

To be successful, you must monitor your body fat levels. Depending on the program, I recommend that everyone take measurements of his or her body fat levels every 1-2 weeks. This is essential. The only way to know if your mass or fat loss program is successful is by monitoring your measurements, weight and body fat levels.

For example, I was recently on a fat loss diet, and I did not lose any weight for three weeks. At first I thought that I needed to drop my calories further because the current levels were not working for me. I did not want to do this because as a hardgainer, dropping my calories too low can result in too much muscle loss.

So, before I committed to a more drastic diet, I checked my body fat records, which I take every 1-2 weeks. Was I in for a shock. According to my body fat calculations I was actually getting leaner. Even though my weight did not change during that three-week period, my body fat levels went down 3%! Since I did not lose any weight during that time, the fat must have been replaced by muscle. I would have never known this by simply looking in the mirror.

Another example is last year when I was on a mass cycle. I was eating a tremendous amount of calories and gaining weight like crazy. I stopped the diet once I began to notice that my fat gains were larger than my muscle gains. I would never have noticed this if I had not closely monitored my body fat levels. I expect to gain some fat on a mass diet, but I always want to gain more muscle than fat. If I had not kept track of my body fat levels, I would have gained too much fat.

There are many methods of measuring your body fat and some are quite expensive. While many consider underwater weighing to be the most accurate, no method is 100% precise — they all have some margin of error. It's not important to know the exact number — **what's important is to use the same method each time you take your measurements so you can have a consistent record of your progress.** I just use an inexpensive skin fold caliper. They cost anywhere from $12-$40 and are simple to use.

A good caliper is essential. Without it, you won't know how exactly your body is responding to your diet and training routine. Just looking in the mirror and guessing is not acceptable. If you want to start getting great results, you must develop the habit of accurately tracking your progress. If you don't, you will continue to go in circles. This may seem like a "hassle", but nothing worth having is ever easy to attain.

Intermediate and advanced fat loss techniques

The secret to increased fat loss

Ok, so you just got started on a program of walking or light cardio and some basic lifting, maybe some dumbbell work, nothing fancy. You feel better, you've lost a few pounds, you have more energy and you're confident that you're getting healthier.

But you want more

You want the results to come faster. You want to look in the mirror and really SEE the difference. You want other people to see the difference too. You want more than "a little tone." Maybe you want a nice hard chiseled six-pack with a small waist, or maybe streamlined, muscular thighs. Well, if you're prepared to step up to the next level and pay the price necessary to reach the next rung on the ladder, here's how you do it.

The answer is very, very simple. As you leave the novice stage behind, it's time to start working harder. That's it! Were you expecting something more esoteric? Some secret Bulgarian periodization program and thermogenic / anabolic supplement stack? Sorry, but the secret is that there is no secret. A great body all boils down to outright effort and hard work. Not counting the genetic freaks that seem to have been born with muscles and zero fat, there's one thing that all people with great bodies have in common: they all work HARD, HARD, HARD!

If you want to ascend beyond the lowly beginner level you simply have to push yourself harder. When you're pushing yourself out of the comfort zone, it hurts. Frankly, sometimes it sucks! But outside the comfort zone is where you grow. Staying inside the comfort zone will only maintain you at best but usually it sends you plummeting into a downward spiral. Most people retreat back into the confines of their comfort zone the minute the effort gets difficult. The comfort zone is a very dangerous place because if you slide back into the comfort zone even once, then it starts becoming a habit.

First, it's stopping just a few minutes short on your cardio or coasting on level 5 when you could be doing level 7. Then you start blowing off workouts completely. Pretty soon, you're sliding back in other areas of your life, you slide back from spending quality time with your family, and you slide back from saving money and watching your finances. You become a backslider!

You can either be a backslider or you can be an achiever but you can't be both and you can't "hang out" in between; it's one or the other. Although you might think you're safe just maintaining in the comfort zone, unbeknownst to you, you are always in motion in either a forward or a backward direction. There's no such thing as standing still.

The achiever is the person who is aware that to "stand still inside the comfort zone" is akin to dying, so he or she is always moving forward. The only way to move forward is with hard work and effort in the direction of a specific goal.

Absolutely, positively do not waste your money on gimmicks

Once you begin getting a taste of what real hard training is like, it often becomes tempting to succumb to the error of looking for the "easy way." An electrode on your abs, a "fat-melting" cream, a pill, a drink mix, a drug. Anything and everything except sweat and hard work. But **shortcuts will always fail you in the long run.**

You are setting yourself up for so much trouble if you give in to the lure of the quick fix. You see, it's all about the Law of Sowing and Reaping. This great law of life states that your rewards can only come back to you in direct proportion to what you put in. Everything has its price and that price must be paid in advance.

If you were a farmer, how ridiculous would it be for you to skip the planting of the seeds in the spring and then go out in the fields looking for a harvest in the fall? How ridiculous would it be to stand in front of a wood burning stove and say: "Ok stove, give me some heat and then I'll put in some wood."

But isn't it the same thing when you take a pill or attach some electrodes to your stomach, or smear some cream on your thighs and expect to lose the flab without exercise or eating right? Even if you've made the decision to avoid gimmicks, in today's marketplace, how do you know what a gimmick is and what's legit? After all, these marketing people are smart; they know how to play on your emotions and make gimmicks sound scientific. Don't feel bad; judging by the e-mails I get every day, most other people don't know the difference either. Nearly all of these e-mails include this sentence: Does "it" work?

Here's how to tell if "it" is a gimmick or not: If it makes getting in phenomenal shape sound easy and effortless, then it's a gimmick. If it addresses the symptom but not the cause, it's a gimmick. If your gut feeling says it sounds too good to be true, it's a gimmick. If it looks like a duck, walks like a duck and quacks like a duck, it's a duck! Do yourself a favor and stop looking for a quick ride to the top.

Double your rate of fat loss in the next 7 days

How would you like to learn a way to double your fat loss in the next seven days? I know, I know - sounds like a gimmick, right? Well, it's not! It's really quite simple. To burn more fat you have to burn more calories. Most beginners start off with three days a week of cardio training. Usually they see some results initially because their bodies aren't accustomed to exercise and any increase in activity above no activity will always produce some results.

More often than not, the results begin to slow down a bit within a few months of training. Then they scratch their heads and wonder why it's not working anymore. This is why: Because three days a week is for beginners, and you're no longer a beginner. **If you want twice as much fat loss and you want it twice as fast, double your cardio.**

Suppose you burn 400 calories per workout for three workouts per week. That's a total of 1200 calories per week burned. If you doubled that to six days per week at 400 calories per workout, you would burn 2400 calories. YOU JUST DOUBLED YOUR FAT LOSS EVERY WEEK! That was a real no-brainer, wasn't it?

Triple your rate of fat loss in the next 7 days

While we're on the subject of burning more calories, what would happen if, in addition to increasing your cardio from three to six days per week, you increased the intensity so that you are burning 600 calories per workout? With six workouts at 600 calories per workout you're up to 3600 calories per week. YOU JUST TRIPLED YOUR FAT LOSS! Yes it's that simple and the solution was right there in front of you all along. By the way, this kind of frequent cardio is how people reach 3 - 4% body fat for competitions: MINIMIUM six days per week of HARD cardio, 45 minutes per session.

<u>Main points for losing fat AND building muscle</u>

High-intensity for bodybuilding involves the application of maximum effort to build maximum muscle in minimum time. High-intensity training bodybuilders don't waste energy trying out the latest super routines in the muscle magazines. They don't train "instinctively." They generally don't squander training times with pumping exercises. They don't adopt the attitude that performing a few extra sets will make up for earlier sets that were poorly executed.

Instead, successful high-intensity training bodybuilders focus mostly on compound exercises such as the dead lift, squat, bent over row, leg press, and other heavy movements. These bodybuilders endeavor to gradually build their poundages by adding a repetition or so each workout and/or increasing the weight by small increments as often as possible, because they know that **getting stronger on the big movements is the best way to stimulate real gains in size.** They know exactly what exercises and weights they are going to use when they arrive at the gym. They strive to get the most out of every repetition and every set.

High-intensity training bodybuilding comprises the soundest application of the principles of exercise physiology. It's a methodical, disciplined, uncomplicated approach to physique development. If you are a drug-free trainee interested in maximizing your natural bodybuilding potential, **high-intensity training is the fastest route to your destination.**

<u>Keep volume low and intensity high</u>

Some claim that you must do a certain number of sets per body part to induce muscular growth. While it's true that the volume of work performed is a consideration, if volume were the primary stimulus for growth then marathon runners would have massively muscle legs. Instead, a casual observation of distance runners almost always reveals thin legs that appear nearly devoid of appreciable muscle.

Intensity that is, the amount of effort applied to each set, supersedes volume when it comes to producing results. Coupled with the gradual progression in poundage, intensity is the key to growth. In fact, one set performed at 100 percent intensity is far more productive than 10 sets performed at 75 percent intensity.

100 percent intensity means performing a set until you are unable, despite your most aggressive effort, to squeeze out one more repetition with good form. This is also known as training to muscle fatigue or failure. It is simple in concept but difficult in execution. Most trainees who think that they are training to fatigue actually terminate their sets well before reaching true fatigue, particularly when it comes to heavy leg exercises. The mind gives out before the body.

High-intensity training bodybuilding is based upon the notion that muscular growth is the result of the body's effort to protect itself from the stress of training heavy. **The more intense the stress, the greater the body's protective response.** This is why the highest possible intensity, taking each work set to the point of muscular fatigue, is required for the fastest progress.

Pushing each set to muscular failure is the most efficient way to train because it ensures the greatest numbers of muscle fibers are stimulated within the shortest amount of time and with the lowest possible volume of work. The all-or-none principle of muscle fiber recruitment states that a muscle uses only the minimum number of fibers necessary to complete a given task and that those fibers contract with maximal force. As you proceed through a set, the muscle fibers that initially lifted the weight become fatigued, forcing fresh fibers to assist in continuing the set. By the time you reach muscular fatigue, most or all of the target muscle fibers have been exhausted. Training to fatigue also ensures that you use the heaviest possible weight for the given number of repetitions. Both of these scenarios set the stage for the fastest possible growth.

This begs the question: if one set to fatigue is good, aren't two sets better and 10 sets better still? No. Performing an excessive number of sets of the given exercise will not increase intensity, it increases volume. It's essential to understand that the body possesses a limited ability to cope with the demands of any stressor, including exercise. **The right amount of high-intensity training leads to results; too much high-intensity training leads to overtraining.** Needless to say, muscular growth will not occur in an overtrained body.

Train briefly and infrequently

Once you understand that training as hard as possible ensures maximum growth stimulation, the next point to grasp is that training as briefly as possible ensures the body has the resources it needs to provide growth. Bear in mind that the body's first priority after a workout is to recover the energy expended during that workout. Only after the body returns to its pre-workout state will it begin the process of supercompensation or growth. It stands to reason that trainees should **perform the minimum amount of work required to stimulate growth to preserve enough energy to foster the growth process.**

There exists no ideal workout length or set. These parameters vary among trainees, depending upon the individual genetic makeup, training history, and lifestyle. But it's safe to say that if you're training in proper high-intensity training style, one or two sets of any exercise is plenty, with six sets being the maximum one should perform for any single body part. Less is probably better for most people.

In general, two workouts per week or a workout every three to four days is sufficient for most to make progress. This applies to advanced trainees as well as beginners. In fact, advanced trainees may need to workout even less often than beginners because their increased strength and ability to generate more effort places their bodies under greater stress. Whatever frequency you initially choose, you should **add more rest days between your workouts if you find that you're still tired and sore by the time of your next workout** or if you fail to increase poundages/repetitions regularly.

Train for strength

Imagine that you currently bench press a maximum of 250 pounds for eight repetitions. You spend the next 12 months performing continuous tension, muscle confusion, and other alleged muscle building techniques. At the end of the twelve-month period, you can still bench press a maximum of 250 pounds for eight repetitions. How much muscle to think you'll have gained? The answer is none. Yes, none, even after years worth of effort.

That's because a relationship exists between the muscle strength and its size. Sadly, many trainees never comprehend this reality. Instead of making a conscious effort to increase their poundages regularly, they fall into the trap of trying every new technique glorified in the bodybuilding magazines. But because they don't get stronger, they don't get bigger.

Don't be swayed by the throng of so-called bodybuilders who perform set after set of an exercise with the goal of achieving a maximum pump. **A pump has nothing to do with true growth; it is merely a temporary state in which the muscle is engorged with blood.**

If you want to build real, lasting muscle tissue, you must make the muscle stronger. This means training for strength. When you're able to do the target number of repetitions with the given weight, it's time to increase that weight. This increase should be small, about five to ten pounds for leg exercises and 2 1/2 to five pounds on upper body exercises is usually enough.

Most people, when they even bother to increase their weights, make the mistake of increasing them too much. This leads to a rapid deterioration of form. Don't be impatient; overtime, small increases add up to a large increase.

Use an appropriate repetition range

Many authorities believe that hypertrophy can be maximized by repetitions in the range of about 8 to 12. This is a useful principle to follow but, in truth, there can be a significant difference in productive repetition ranges among individuals and among body parts within the same individual.

In general, sets of about five repetitions or less should be avoided by bodybuilders because such low repetitions demonstrate strength rather than build it. In addition, sets of about five repetitions or less at a typical cadence heavily stress the joints and connective tissue without keeping the muscle fibers loaded long enough to provoke growth. Sets of about 15 repetitions or more promote greater metabolic and muscular endurance adaptations rather than strength/growth. **This leaves a usable repetition range for bodybuilding purposes of about 6 to 15.**

A compelling amount of evidence suggests that the lower body responds better than the upper body to higher repetition ranges. As such, it may be best use about 10 to 15 repetitions for lower body work and about 6 to 10 repetitions for upper body work. Experiment with both the upper and lower end of these repetition ranges to discover what works best for you.

Focus on the major muscle groups

If you want to get bigger, you are going to have to pay the price in the form of agonizing effort on exercises that allow you to use relatively heavy weights. The focus should be on compound movements that works several muscle groups at the same time, such as the squat, deadlifts, chin up, bent over row, and bench press. In fact, a very productive routine that stimulates serious growth from head to toe can be built around just these five exercises.

That's not to say that calf raises, arm exercises, and abdominal work should be avoided. They can be part of your program, especially once you're an advanced trainee. Just understand that you'll simulate more biceps growth by doing heavy chin-ups and rows than you will by doing set after set of concentration curls.

The majority of the muscle mass on your body is found in your hips, legs, back, and chest. The only way to gain the pounds of muscular body weight that will accentuate your appearance is by increasing the size of these muscles. **Train the large muscle groups heavy and hard and the smaller groups will gain as well.**

Use proper training style and technique

For best results, it's not enough to lift heavy weights, you must lift them properly. Heaving, thrusting, jerking, and bouncing should be avoided at all costs. As a bodybuilder, your mission in the gym is to exhaust your muscles so that they are forced to rebuild larger and stronger. Weights and machines are the tools you used for that purpose. While you want to lift as much weight as possible for given number of repetitions, you want to do so within the context of proper form.

Jerky and bouncing motions may allow you to lift more weight than you otherwise might be able to handle but such motions minimize the load on the muscles you are trying to work. **Such motions also multiply the stress on your joints and connective tissue, setting you up for injury.**

Some training authorities suggest following a 2 to 4 protocol in which the positive motion takes two seconds in the negative motion takes four seconds. This is fine general advice but what's important to remember is that you want to keep the muscle loaded throughout the entire repetition. Lift the weight with power, precision, and focus; pause for second in the fully contracted position; and lower the weight reasonably slowly while feeling the muscle resist the weight all the way down.

Emphasize recovery more than you think you should

Training provides the stimulus for growth but the growth process does not take place while you train. It takes place later when you rest and especially when you sleep.

Taking an adequate number of days off between workouts is only part of the recovery equation. You must also ensure that your rest days are truly rest days. **If your goal is to add substantial muscle to your frame, minimize your activity level outside the gym.** Playing full-court basketball may be fun but doing so regularly will deplete energy that would otherwise be directed toward recovery and supercompensation. Determine your priorities and act accordingly.

Nor can you afford to frolic until the wee hours of the morning if your dream is to get big. Sleep is critical to the growth process and must not be overlooked. Six hours a night is the bare minimum you should sleep and seven or eight hours is preferable. **Understand that even the most painstakingly devised and religiously followed training program will yield little or no gains if you're sleep deprived.**

Eat well and often

If training serves as the catalyst for growth and sleep provides the opportunity for growth, and food provides the raw materials required for growth.

The ideal eating plan to get big is based around lean protein sources (lean beef, chicken breast, turkey breast, fish, egg whites, and low-fat dairy products), complex carbohydrates (oatmeal, brown rice, yams, and potatoes), fibrous carbohydrates (vegetables and whole fruits), and a small to moderate amount of healthy fats (egg yolks, vegetable oils, nuts, and nut butters). The occasional addition, perhaps a few times weekly, of sweets and fast foods is fine, but keep in mind that a steady intake of sugar and fat laden foods can lead to a rapid accumulation of body fat.

Structure your eating plan to provide five to seven moderate size meals each day. **Smaller, more frequent feedings provide your muscles with a constant supply of the nutrients** they need for growth without promoting excessive fat storage. Such an eating plan will keep your energy level stable and minimize cravings.

Supplements such as protein powers and meal replacements should be viewed as conveniences rather than necessities. Natural food should form the cornerstones of your nutrition program, but when time is short a meal replacement or protein drink is preferable to fast food or no food.

Combine machines and free weights

The arguments in supporting both free weights and machines are loud and long. Free weight supporters claim that the balance required to lift free weights provide a stronger growth stimulus to the muscles and machine lovers point out that machine users can work their muscles harder precisely because they don't have to balance the weight. Free weights are said to be a more natural form of resistance while machines are designed to make up for the inherent shortcomings of barbells and dumbbells.

Each side as valid arguments, so why not get the benefits of both by combining free weights and machines in your program? A very productive routine can be designed around barbells, dumbbells, and whatever machines you have access to.

Keep a daily workout record

Most trainees have no idea where they're going to reach their destination because they don't keep track of where they've been. That is, they don't keep a training diary.

To make the most out of high-intensity bodybuilding, you're going to have to keep records. Don't trust your memory; put your performances on paper. For every work set completed, you should write down the weights used and repetitions obtained. Refer to your training diary during your next training session and try as hard as possible to better your previous performance.

This implies, of course, that the only frequent changes in your routine should be in repetitions and poundages, not exercises. While some variety is reasonable, continually changing exercises doesn't give you the benefit of establishing linear progression from workout to workout, which is the basis for long-term improvement. This does not mean you should use the same exercises for years on end. It only means that you should stick with a given exercise until it ceases to work for you. Leave the so-called instinctive training principle, which states that one should "confuse" the muscles by constantly changing exercises from workout to workout, for those who are more interested in being a Poser than in making progress.

Diet to obtain muscular definition and low bodyfat

While getting bigger is the primary goal of the typical trainee, most serious bodybuilders eventually develop the urge to improve their muscular definition. After all, the source of the unique appearance of bodybuilders, the thing that distinguishes them from just another big person who pumps iron is crisp, sharply delineated musculature.

In truth, training for definition is a fallacy. **Definition is not a quality that can be trained into a muscle; it is nothing more than the absence of fat over a well-developed muscle.** The peaks, valleys, separations, and veins that characterize a detailed physique exist in anyone who has developed a respectable degree of muscle mass. If these muscular details cannot be seen, it's because they are obscured by bodyfat.

The best way to train for definition is to adopt a sensible fat loss plan. Put simply, you'll have to eat less. But you want to eat only a little less, starvation diets burn more muscle than fat. A slight reduction, perhaps 300 to 400 calories daily, should be sufficient to set the fat loss machinery in motion. Aim for a loss of just one pound weekly; more rapid weight loss will quickly eat into your hard earned muscle mass.

The best fat loss diets are based around frequent feedings. Eat five to seven small meals a day consisting of lean protein, a moderate amount of carbohydrates, and a small model fat. While mainstream nutritionists typically promote high carbohydrate eating plans, many competitive bodybuilders find that they get their best fat loss results by consuming a moderate amount of carbohydrates, perhaps 40 percent or less of their calories. These bodybuilders also find a better to taper their carbohydrates as the day goes on by eating starchy carbohydrates for breakfast and lunch and fibrous carbohydrates such as broccoli, a staple source of carbohydrates for bodybuilders, during the late afternoon in the evening.

A moderate amount of cardiovascular activity can assist in fat loss. Whether you choose to run or walk at a fast pace outdoors or indoors on a treadmill, or bike indoors or outdoors, or use one of the numerous cardio machines available at commercial gyms. **Start out by performing the activity two or three times weekly for 20 minutes at a moderate intensity.** Gradually increase the duration and number of cardio sessions. Since excessive cardiovascular work can cut into muscle size, perform the minimum amount of cardio activity required to keep fat loss occurring until you reach her goal. Try not to exceed five 45-minute cardio sessions weekly.

While trying to get lean, your approach to weight training should be the same as when you're striving to add mass: train intensely, briefly, and infrequently. At this point, increasing your volume is an even bigger mistake than it was when you training for size, as a decrease in caloric intake and the inclusion of cardio work makes you more susceptible to overtraining.

What about developing an impressive "six-pack" abdominal region? This again is a matter of eliminating excess body fat through diet and cardio. Performing countless crunches, setups, and leg raises in hopes of bringing out the abs is a waste of time and effort. As your percentage of body fat lowers, your abs will become more prominent. **To display a truly impressive rock hard mid-section, you'll need to lower your percentage of body fat too well under 10 percent**, and undertaking that requires discipline and diligence. **Women would need to drop their percentage of body fat to the low teens.**

Questions and answers

I get bombarded with e-mails from all over the world, from Japan to Argentina, and it's interesting to see how small differences there are, really. Everybody wants to know how to get stronger and more buff. Everybody wants to lose bodyfat. Everybody wants to know if protein drinks really work. The last question is a simple "yes," but the two before that are little bit trickier.

Still, there are some more specific questions that inevitably pop up from time to time. Here are a few of them.

Q: My friend has really peaked biceps while mine are not, while we both curl the same weight. How come? What can I do to increase my peak?

A: Unfortunately, the shape of muscle is largely determined by genetics, so blame mom and dad. However, there are some things you can do. The biceps consists of two separate heads, and by smart training you can develop both to their limit. Don't expect to be able to solely pinpoint one of the two, but you can shift the focus a little. One exercise I have found particularly well for bringing out the peak is bicep curls with a straight barbell, where you hold the bar with a more-than-shoulder-width grip and tuck in your elbows against your sides. Experiment a little to see what works best for you. Start with slightly less weight than usual and do 12-15 reps just to feel where the burn materializes. Then flex your biceps in a classic bicep-pose and use your other hand to squeeze the peak of your biceps. If that's where the lactic acid burn is at, you've found an exercise that will work.

Q: I have a horrible sweet tooth, but I need to get in shape. What can I do to avoid going crazy?

A: Use the window of opportunity immediately after your workouts to have a handful or two of candy. As I've talked about before, that is the one time when you should be eating something sugary to get your body back into an anabolic state again. Make sure to get something sugary though, not fat. Fat has a lot more calories per gram than sugar, and fat will slow down the release of the sugars into your blood stream. Examples of good candy: Jelly beans, sugar babies and reduced fat cookies. Examples of bad candy: Chocolate, candy bars and peanut-butter cups.

Q: You say I should do lat pulldowns to the front rather than behind the neck. Why?

A: To work the lats effectively, you must keep your back slightly arched. By pulling the bar to the front, you're all but guaranteed to keep the arch, while a pull behind the neck lends itself to cheating as you get tired. Thereby you could routinely rob yourself of the benefit from the last few reps of each set without even knowing it. In addition, it's a more natural movement to pull the bar to the front. Your shoulders are at less of a vulnerable angle, and as you get stronger you might avoid cumulative shoulder injuries. This is only true for some people, but the bad news is that you usually don't know if you're one of them until it's too late, so play it safe and assume that you are.

Last but not least, there is an important thing to notice about the lat pulls to the front. You might be tempted to lean back too much when you get tired, thus giving yourself an extra pull. Try to avoid this kind of swaying - sit upright with a lightly arched back, and stay that way throughout the exercise.

Q: What are your thoughts on sports drinks such as Gatorade, Hydra Fuel and such?

A: I don't have any problem with them as long as they're consumed in conjunction with hard and prolonged exercise. Most sports drinks are full of sugar and are formulated to replace lost fluid through sweating, so they're not suitable for drinking with your dinner. In the gym or on a field, they're perfectly fine. Just watch for artificial ingredients. If the drink has a long laundry-list of suspicious-sounding chemicals that you can't even pronounce, pick something else.

Q: My friend is considering buying some steroids, but is concerned about getting ripped off rather than getting the real thing. Is there any web site that can help you identify the legit labels and such?

A: Uh-huh. And I bet your "friend" is about your age and height too, right? Look, here's another reason not to take steroids: It's virtually impossible to know what you're taking. If the crook peddling this dope fills a vial with liquid cleaning agent and slaps a realistic-looking sticker on it, you wouldn't have a clue of what you injected until you woke up in the E.R. If you're lucky, that is. I've seen sites where they promise to show you the telltale signs of counterfeit labels, but guess what? The counterfeiters read the same advice! The bottom line is that all you have to go on is the word of the seller, and, quite frankly, do you think he cares more about your health than his own wallet? Really?

Q: I just can't seem to hit my rear delts properly, and that is getting more and more of a problem as my side and front delts grow. What can I do?

A: Try attaching a handle to the lower pulley on a pulley machine. Then kneel on the floor with your side turned to the pulley. Grab the handle with the hand furthest away from the pulley and lean forward so that you support your upper body with your free hand against the floor. Let the handle pull your other arm so that you feel a good stretch in the rear delt. In other words, if you got your right side facing the pulley, you hold the handle in your left hand while supporting yourself with the right hand on the floor. You should be so far away from the pulley machine that you have resistance even at your most stretched. Then simply pull the handle out to the side as far you can without moving or swaying the rest of your body. The only thing moving should be your shoulder and your arm. This way you can experiment with different angles and slight variations to hit the rear delts 100%.

Q: How important is warm-up, really? I know I'm supposed to do at least 5 minutes on the bike before I hit the weights, but I have very little time…

A: Let me put it this way: If you can "afford" 5 minutes more of watching TV, or 5 minutes of dozing after lunch, or whatever, you'd be better off spending those 5 minutes on a warm-up. Not only do you get your body going so that it utilizes fat for fuel better, it also drastically decreases your risk of injury - especially if you're planning on lifting big. There's no justification for skipping something that can do so much for your health and safety, unless you're a top-level executive who sleeps 3 hours per night and makes 15-minute appointments to play with your kids on the weekends. If you're a mere mortal like the rest of us, who spends a few hours in front of the tube now and then, you're making an active choice to watch TV instead of looking out for yourself. And by the way, don't you think a single torn muscle, with all the handicaps and rehab it involves, makes up for the time you'd save by skipping the warm-up during your entire life? Play it safe - always warm up.

Q: How come the people in before and after-pictures in the ads always look so much better than I do, no matter how hard I work out, diet, and take the supplements they push?

A: And drinking certain brands of soda doesn't make you an extreme-sporting mega hunk either, even if their ad implies so. Read the fine print. There's always a puny little disclaimer saying something to the effect of: "Mr. Ripped on the picture experienced exceptional results. The typical user may not expect similar results." In plain English, that means they all but admit that while the dude on a picture is a nice fairy tale, the Muscle Fairy will most likely visit not you. The sad truth is that there are no shortcuts. When an ad claims that their product is 3,463% better than the competition, it does not mean you'll gain muscle 3,463% faster. In fact, most scientific claims I've seen are taken out of context. Sure, a certain ingredient in product X may do a lot of good for an 80-year old female diabetic, or help an obese lab rat, but to expect even remotely the same results in a 230 lb, 25-year old male bodybuilder is ridiculous. Yet, they can quote the scientific study and advertise it to create the illusion that the 80-year old woman figures somehow applies to you. It's dirty, but it works. Otherwise they wouldn't keep doing it. Of course, there are honest facts in ads, and there are reputable companies who don't try to scam you with inflated claims, but it's generally easy to spot the difference. Remember: If something sounds too good to be true, it usually is.

Q: I have kind of an embarrassing problem… I don't use steroids, and still I've noticed my pecs are kind of "drooping" when relaxed, making them look like the beginning stages of breasts. I train religiously, I have very little bodyfat, and still I think it keeps getting worse! What's up with this??

A: Don't panic. What you're seeing is probably the effect of too much decline bench pressing. Lately, I've seen a surge the number of people using decline presses, the kind where you lock your legs between two rolls and lay with your head down on a declining bench. This often allows you to use slightly more weight in the bench press, which as we all know is the Holy Grail for 99% of the male gym rats ages 15 to 30. The bad news is; the pectoralis major has a fan-shape, allowing you to train different areas to different degrees. If you do a lot of incline presses, you're weaker compared to the flat press, but you train the upper part of your chest. This gives you a well-balanced, rock-solid look. However, if you train the lower part of your pecs too much, especially if neglecting the upper part, you grow the muscles into looking like a flat-chested dude with beginning bitch tits. Make sense? The muscles will grow according to how you train them, so my advice to you is to stop doing decline presses immediately, and focus on flat and incline presses for a couple of months. When you've balanced out and start feeling comfortable again, you can go back to a normal training routine again - splitting the focus equally between the upper and lower part of the chest.

Q: Why is breakfast so important?

A: When you've been asleep for 8 or so hours, you haven't eaten for at least 8 hours, possibly more like 10 or 11 hours. This means your body is really low on amino acids and carbs, both something you want to have floating around in your body to stay anabolic. The best way to break the starvation of your muscles is to have a hearty breakfast as soon as possible as you wake up. Also, if you work out early in the day, it's extra important to get a lot of carbs with your breakfast, as you'll need it to fuel your workout.

Q: What is the best repetition range for building muscle?

A: At an average repetition cadence (speed), generally 8 -12 reps per set will elicit the greatest gains in lean mass. Sets consisting of less than 6 or 8 reps generally focus on muscle strength, whereas a high number of reps each set targets muscle endurance.

Detailed Answer:

The conventional view that fewer reps in each set equates to more muscle gain is a bit too simplistic. In reality, when one performs sets with very high weight and low reps, the main physiological change is a strengthening of neuromuscular pathways. In other words, high weight/low reps strengthen the brain's ability to activate muscle. However, if we bump up the reps slightly while decreasing the weight as necessary, the muscle tissue will perform more total work, and thus more muscle growth will occur. However, if the reps are increased too high, the main effect will be an increase in muscle endurance.

Through research, it has been determined that the best range for hypertrophy (muscle gain) is roughly between 8-12 reps. As the reps are decreased from this range, the program will elicit greater strength gains will less size. In contrast, more than 12 reps mainly allows for increases in muscular endurance.

Q: Does weight training cause high blood pressure?

A: Natural bodybuilders are among the most fit individuals in athletics. While weight training itself has little effect on cardiovascular health, it does not increase blood pressure in the long term. Although blood pressure does rise during any type of exercise, which is not dangerous for healthy individuals. However, most bodybuilders also engage in cardiovascular exercise, which is well established for decreasing blood pressure.

Also, natural bodybuilders tend to be very lean; not only on the "outside," but also on the "inside," as they tend to have less fatty plaque lining artery walls, and are therefore at a reduced risk for atherosclerosis. Further, the "large heart syndrome" that many purport as a result of weight training has not been proven in research.

Q: Is it possible to gain muscle strength or muscle endurance without gaining muscle size?

A: It is possible to gain strength without increasing muscle size (hypertrophy). Similarly, it is possible to enhance muscle endurance without hypertrophy. However, it may be difficult to train for both goals at the same time.

- Training for muscle endurance is generally achieved through high repetitions and lighter weights.

- To train for strength while minimizing gains in muscle mass, it is advisable to perform low repetitions per set, using explosive movements (short concentric contractions) while lowering the weights under control. Be sure to be adequately warmed up before starting into the working sets.

Detailed Answer:

Training for strength over size is largely attained through manipulating the neuromuscular system (brain-muscle connection); that is, strengthening the nervous system as a muscle "activator". As a protective mechanism for the body, the central nervous system has safeguards in place that shut down muscle activity when the muscle attempts to work at too high an intensity.

Specifically, one of these systems works through an organelle found in tendons of muscle, which shuts down muscle activity when it senses that there is too much strain on a muscle. Also, for the untrained individual (or somebody who rarely lifts very heavy weights), the connection between muscle and brain may be relatively weak. To train the neuromuscular connection, it is advisable to perform low repetitions per set, using explosive movements (short concentric contractions) while lowering the weights under control.

Be sure to be adequately warmed up before starting into the working sets. Although muscle fiber density may increase from this type of training, hypertrophy is minimized since high resistance/low rep training does not elicit changes in extra-fibril structures (blood vessels, organelles like mitochondria). At the same time, strength gains will be evident through neuromuscular manipulation.

Training for muscle endurance is generally achieved through high repetitions and lighter weights. With this type of training, the major change to the muscle is the ability to manage metabolic waste, and fuel utilization. For example, the muscle is better able to utilize lactate as a fuel rather than allow it to minimize muscle performance.

Also, more efficient fuel sources such as fats make up a larger portion of the muscle's fuel. Rather than carbohydrates which tend to promote metabolic waste accumulation. Note, however, that some of these changes include increased capillary (and blood vessel) density and mitochondria, changes that reduce muscle density. Nevertheless, these changes will not cause a significant increase in muscle size.

Since these two goals require quite different methods of training, a good approach may be to periodize your training. That is, train for muscle endurance for 3-4 weeks, and then switch to a training program geared towards building muscle strength.

Q: What is meant by the term Basal Metabolic Rate?

A: Basal Metabolic Rate (BMR) or basal metabolism represents the minimal energy expended to keep a resting, awake body alive. This requires about 60-70% of the total energy use by the body. The processes involved include maintaining a heartbeat, respiration, temperature and other functions. It does not include energy used for physical activity or digesting foods. Basal metabolism accounts for roughly 1 kcalorie/kilogram (2.2 lbs.)/hour. I use the term 'roughly," due to the fact that the amount of energy used for basal metabolism depends primarily upon lean body mass.

Q: What causes delayed onset muscle soreness?

A: The cause for delayed onset muscle soreness (DOMS) has been debated at length by exercise physiologists, and is still not fully understood. Mechanisms for theories proposed in the past have included lactic acid buildup, torn tissue, muscle spasm, and connective tissue damage. Of these, the lactic acid buildup theory, and spasm theory have largely been discounted by exercise physiologists. Currently, the most accepted theory for DOMS seems to be muscle/connective tissue damage due to mechanical forces on the muscle and connective tissue.

Q: I heard that exercising on an empty stomach leads to losses in lean body mass. Should I really be exercising on an empty stomach?

A: There are benefits to working out on an empty stomach, and different benefits when one works out after eating. Ultimately, one should choose the method based on their fitness goals. As a rule of thumb, it may be best to perform workouts on an empty stomach if one's main goal is bodyfat loss. However, if one is only concerned with gaining lean mass, eating 30-60 minutes before a workout may be a good idea.

For people looking to lose bodyfat while increasing muscle mass at the same time, it may be best to take advantage of the key benefits of each method. For example, one could try working out on an empty stomach some days, and eat 30-60 minutes before working out on other days (i.e. eat before resistance exercise sessions; do not eat before cardio). Following is a detailed breakdown of the benefits and drawbacks to each method:

Eating 30-60 minutes before a Workout

Benefits:

- Maximizes liver and muscle glycogen, a fuel stored in muscle that is necessary for intense exercise (assuming that the meal is balanced).

- Prevents the breakdown of muscle tissue (by preventing the secretion of the hormone cortisol).

- Allows for longer duration workouts.

- May increase secretion of growth hormone (particularly with exercise that elicits high lactate production, like intense cardio) therefore greater utilization of fat as fuel, free fatty acid (FFA) release, and protein synthesis.

Drawbacks:

- Suppresses FFA release from fat stores (due to the presence of insulin).

- Excess insulin (which easily occurs through eating too many calories or high glycemic foods) may cause hypoglycemia, leading to depleted muscle glycogen stores therefore exerciser "crashes".

Exercise on Empty Stomach

Benefits:

- Increases FFA availability in blood therefore increases the amount fats burned as energy.

- May increase secretion of growth hormone (particularly with exercise that elicits high lactate production, like intense cardio) therefore greater utilization of fat as fuel,

FFA release, and protein synthesis (note that this is an unresolved issue, as it contradicts the bullet above).

Drawbacks:

• Increased production of cortisol therefore leads to the breakdown of muscle tissue.

Q: On certain training days such as when I do back and biceps together, sometimes it is difficult to hold onto the bar because of forearm fatigue. Is there anything I can do to correct this?

A: Forearm strength is often a limiting factor, especially when handling heavy weights vertically such as pull-ups or deadlift. Chalk, sticky pads, or weightlifting straps can help with handling the load when necessary, however, as a rule of thumb, it is best to work through this discomfort since these very activities are some of the best exercises for developing the forearms and building grip strength. On the contrary, straps and chalk should always be used.

When to use straps and chalk:

1. Your ability to hold the weight compromises the safety of the movement, or

2. Lack of grip strength limits your ability to strengthen/develop the target muscle effectively.

Q: I have had a cold the past couple of days and was wondering if it is a good idea to still exercise?

A: You may think it is a good idea not to engage in vigorous exercise when you have the sniffles. However, a new study suggests that if you are well enough to get out of bed, you are probably well enough to get a workout. Researchers at Ball State University in Indiana found that exercising does not delay recovery or worsen symptoms of the common cold.

In the study, 34 moderately fit folks, ages 18-29, were assigned to an exercising group, while 16 additional people of similar age and fitness level were assigned to a non-exercising group. Then both groups were inoculated with a virus to produce upper respiratory illness. The exercising group worked out at 70% of maximum heart rate for 40 minutes per day, every other day.

Researchers collected used facial tissues and administered symptom questionnaires every 12 hours to gauge the progress of the illness and its symptoms. After ten days, analyses of symptoms were similar between the exercising and non-exercising groups. So while you may feel like scaling down your routine if you are feeling under the weather, there seems to be no reason to skip it altogether.

Q: I've heard the terms "concentric and eccentric contractions." What do these mean?

A: A concentric contraction occurs during the lifting phase of an exercise, when the muscle shortens or contracts. For example, when you lift the weight in a bench press, pressing it from your chest to the lock-out position, that is the concentric, or "positive," phase of the exercise. An eccentric contraction occurs during the lowering phase of an exercise, when the muscle lengthens. For example, lowering the weight to your chest during the bench press is the eccentric or "negative," portion of the exercise.

Q: What can I do about 'stretch marks' that appear after I've been weight lifting and gaining size and strength?

A: If you are weight training and gaining some size and muscularity, chances are you will begin to develop stretch marks. This is, to a certain extent, unavoidable. You may minimize their development, however, through the application of a topical antioxidant cream that contains collagen. Regular application of this type of lotion/cream will increase skin elasticity, and thus diminish the formation of stretch marks, but it may not fully prevent their development.

Q: What can I do to prevent muscle cramping?

A: Muscle cramping occurs when a muscle continues to contract, and cannot seem to "let go". The painful sensation one feels is caused by muscle fatigue, and waste products like lactic acid that build up in the muscle. Although the cause of muscle cramps is not entirely understood, a number of factors seem to be involved, including hydration level, electrolyte balance, training history, and chronically tight muscles.

Some factors that may increase muscle cramps:

1. Training history seems to be the most important factor. Exercise beyond an accustomed limit (longer duration, or intensity) will often brings on muscle cramps. However, through regular training, one tends to experience muscle cramps less frequently.

2. Make sure that you are drinking enough water - 10 glasses of water daily (at least 10 oz. each), or if you care to be more precise, 0.6oz/water/lb. of bodyweight. Increase this amount if you consume caffeine. For each cup of coffee, tea, or soda you take in, please be sure to add an additional 10 oz glass of water for each.

3. Through sweating (especially in a hot environment), one tends to lose electrolytes like sodium, potassium, and magnesium. Normally these are replaced in the diet. However, prolonged exercise (longer than 1 hour) in hot environments may create a need for mineral replenishment. Try adding a bit of salt to your foods, and take a multivitamin/mineral supplement and see if this makes a difference.

4. Lastly, tight muscles are best addressed by stretching before and after every workout. Stretching allows more nutrients, blood, etc. into the muscle, and allows you to dispose of waste materials more easily due to increased blood flow.

Q: What is the current theory on using a weight belt? Should I or shouldn't I use one?

A: Weight belts are a handy tool for helping to protect your back on those lifts that may stress it, but that does not mean you should use them on every lift for every rep. When you do an intense exercise that involves the back, such as squats, it would seem logical that you would want that safety precaution in place at all times.

In doing so, however, you may predispose yourself to an injury by taking the muscles that would ordinarily act as natural back supports out of the equation. Essentially, when you are doing a squat, your primary focus in terms of strength is your leg muscles. What most people don't realize is that you are also simultaneously strengthening your back support muscles; abdominals, lower back, obliques, etc.

When you wear a belt, you take those muscles (to a lesser or greater extent depending upon form) out of the chain, and as such they do not get strengthened to the same degree as do your leg muscles. What this may do in the long run is create an imbalance in the body in terms of overall support and equilibrium, which as you continue to grow stronger and use more weight, may increase the risk of injuring yourself in one way or another.

Perhaps the best way of looking at these muscles is to consider them a chain, and as you know, a chain is only as strong as its weakest link. As such, if you're going to strengthen any part of the chain, you better strengthen the whole chain to keep yourself safe and prevent injuries. When would you want to use a belt? Usually, the only time to use a belt is when you are attempting a maximal lift; anywhere from 4 - 6 reps of a challenging weight that involves back support and all-out effort. At all other times, it's a good idea to simply use good form and have a competent spotter on these exercises.

Q: I have been told all of my life that you have to work out at least 30 to 35 minutes in order to begin burning fat. Is there any scientific data you can provide to prove that the 20-minute aerobic solution does in fact burn fat?

A: When trying to lose bodyfat, the duration of the workout is less important than total calorie balance (total calories burned). To lose fat, it is necessary to achieve a calorie deficit. That is, the number of calories you burn must be greater than the number of calories you ingest. Cardiovascular exercise helps you to create this calorie deficit by burning excess calories. Although you can burn calories at any workout intensity, it is most efficient to work at a high-intensity for shorter periods of time compared to long-duration workouts.

For example, working at a high-intensity, one can burn up to 50% more calories in a shorter period of time. More importantly, post workout, you continue to burn calories at an elevated rate up to 142% more than low-intensity aerobics within the first hour following the cardio session. What's more, this elevation in metabolism lasts up to 48 hours post workout, an effect not achieved with low-intensity exercise. The bottom line is that while low-intensity, long-duration exercise is effective for fat loss; typically one sees better results using a high-intensity protocol. Plus, this type of training is more efficient since once spends less time in the gym, but typically experiences better results.

Q: I typically run outdoors, but when it's hot and humid, I head to the treadmill. Does running on the treadmill burn fewer calories?

A: If you're running at speeds under 9 miles an hour (a very fast 6:40-minute-mile pace), treadmill running burns about the same number of calories as running outdoors. But if you run faster than 9 mph, you'll burn fewer calories on the treadmill. The difference can be up to 8 percent because you don't have to overcome wind resistance and because the treadmill belt does propel you along a bit.

Q: A year and a half ago, I started running 5 miles on a treadmill six days a week and lifting weights three times a week. The results have been fabulous; a 74-pound weight loss, a huge drop in blood pressure and an enormous surge in self-esteem. But now my knees ache, especially when I walk downhill. Is this a result of running? What can I do about the pain?

A: Six days a week of high-impact training such as running is very hard on the body, especially the knees. Substituting a low-impact activity such as biking, swimming or the elliptical trainer once or twice a week is much healthier.

Most likely you're experiencing patella-femoral syndrome, also known as pain behind the kneecap. Running, especially on hard surfaces, increases the pressure of the patella (kneecap) on the femur (thighbone) when you bend and straighten your knee.

Q: Is it easier for a man to get six-pack abs than for a woman to?

A: Yes. The appearance of defined, rock-hard ab muscles is possible only if the abs are highly trained and there is very little fat on top of them. On average, women have more total body fat than men, and proportionally they nave more subcutaneous fat. What's more, it's easier for men to lose body fat than it is for women, partly due to hormonal differences. If you put men and women on the same exercise and diet program, men will lose more weight on average. Of course, not every man will lose more fat than every woman will. There are exceptions; some women can achieve a six-pack without tremendous work, and some men have no chance of ever having sleek abs.

The bottom line, don't get frustrated if you can't achieve that six-pack. It may not be a matter of lacking willpower. It could be just a matter of genetic and gender destiny.

Q: I have a friend who does a 5- to 10-minute warm-up on a treadmill, then lifts weights, then does 20 more minutes of cardio. Does her warm-up really count as cardlo? I've heard you need to do 15 consecutive minutes to get benefits.

A: A 5- to 10-minute warm-up certainly would count. Since a warm-up is performed at a low intensity, you won't burn as many calories those first few minutes. But that doesn't mean you're not benefiting. Most people don't need more than two or three minutes to get their heart rate up to the lower end of their target zone. At the lower end of the zone — about 60 percent of your maximum heart rate — your body is working hard enough to achieve health and fitness benefits.

There is no research establishing the minimum number of consecutive minutes necessary to "count," but plenty of research has established the benefits of short cardio bouts.

Of course, if you are training for an endurance event such as a 10k or marathon, 10 minute workouts aren't going to cut it. But for general health and fitness you can break it down, research shows tremendous benefits from performing 15 10-minute exercise bouts per week, including cardio exercise, strength training and stretching.

Q: What happens if I go over my target zone for fat burning?

A: You will burn glycogen (blood glucose), which is fine. The problem, however, is that unless you are a highly trained athlete, you don't have high amounts of glycogen stored in your muscles cells and other storage areas. In this case, cortisol, one of the hormones secreted with exercise begins to break down muscle tissue to transform it into glucose so you can continue to exercise/survive. This process is commonly known as "gluconeogenisis," or the new formation of glucose by breaking down muscle.

Q: Why are strong abdominal muscles so important?

A: A strong mid-section will help support the lower back (lumbar spine). It also helps transfer strength and power from the upper body to the lower. In general, the abdominal muscles, lower back, and pelvic region is called the "core." What you need to strive for is "core stability." When the hip flexor muscles are too tight, it causes inflexibility and forward pelvic tilt. Weak abdominals and a tight lower back will create an excessive arch in the lower back known as "sway back." When an imbalance is present in this area, the result can be pain, poor energy transfer in sports, and general body discomfort. Over time, the result can be spinal segments that lip, spur, and even fuse.

Q: How important is massage therapy to an athlete?

A: In one word "VITAL". Massage does the following: reduces stress, decreases recovery time, promotes healing, increases performance, increases speed, releases toxins and it feels oh, so good! Make sure your massage therapist known your tolerance for pain, what type of massage you've experienced, and your intended benefit from the massage.

Q: Should I stretch before or after I workout with weights?

A: Both. Prior to any stretching, a general warm-up should take place. A bike, rower, treadmill or stepper is fine. This is to heat the body's core temperature. Once the core is warm, perform some moderate intensity stretches. Make certain the entire body is stretched, however spend a little extra time on the specific area you intend on training first. After you finish your lifting routine, you body will be very warm and better able to stretch more deeply. This is the time to gently increase the intensity of your stretching.

Q: If I'm very over weight, should I still lift weights? I don't want to bulk up any more.

A: You absolutely should lift weights. It doesn't need to be your focus, but it needs to be included in your complete program. In most cases, weight training is not cardiovascular in nature. This means your body will not use fat as a primary source of energy while lifting weights. However, weight training does make your body better at consuming calories throughout the day. Because a muscle requires more energy to maintain its structure as compared to fat, your body must use (burn) more calories to maintain that muscles integrity. Aside from all this, if you don't maintain or build muscle as you lose weight, you will become what is known as a "thin, fat person." This is a slightly built person who has no muscle mass.

Q: Is there a difference between types of creatines that are currently available?

A: As some people are aware, you can now find creatine on the market in three forms: phosphate, citrate, and monohydrate. My feeling is that the phosphate variety is not easily absorbed by the body and for this reason will not yield effective and substantial results. The citrate variety seemed to be catching on for a time, but again the research is sketchy here. In fact, nearly all the positive clinical studies that have been done on creatine have utilized the monohydrate form, and this is the only form that I currently recommend.

Q: My doctor told me I am allergic to wheat and dairy products. How could this be? Is there a test or a way to really find out if I am allergic?

A: I think the only way you can find this out is by omitting all forms of those foods from your diet for at least a week, then adding the food back and seeing if your symptoms return. Also, since both wheat and dairy products are found in so many foods, you'll have to read the labels of processed foods especially carefully.

Q: I love chocolate. Is it really bad for you? How much can I eat without sabotaging my healthy eating plan?

A: Chocolate isn't all bad. In fact, chocolate is rich in antioxidants called phenolics, the same compounds in red wine that seem to offer protection against heart disease. And cocoa butter, the fat in chocolate, does not appear to be so bad for your heart and arteries. Its principal saturated fat, stearic acid is converted by the body into oleic acid, a heart-healthy monounsaturated fat also found in olive oil. Pick chocolate made with cocoa butter rather than unhealthy fats such as palm and coconut oils. This means look for cocoa to appear in the ingredients before sugar.

Q: I seem to be addicted to sweets. How do you suggest I stop eating foods high in sugar?

A: Taming your sugar cravings could be a matter of slowly reeducating your tastebuds or learning to feel satisfied with less. If you slowly cut back on sweets, you will find that healthy sweet foods taste exceptionally sweet - fresh strawberries, frozen grapes, mangoes, dried unsweetened cherries. Treats like these will satisfy your sweet tooth if you take the time to eat them with full attention to taste, aroma, and presentation.

Q: What are the pros and cons of eating farm-raised salmon instead of salmon from the wild? I've heard farmed salmon is not a good source of omega-3 fatty acids because of what the fish are fed.

A: I always choose wild salmon over farmed salmon. Flesh from most pen-raised salmon may be lower in beneficial omega-3 fatty acids and higher in harmful saturated fats than that from their wild cousins - a consequence of what they are fed. And worst of all, is that the under exercised muscles of salmon reared in cages produce a soft, bland-tasting fish that just doesn't stand up to the wild version. The product label will tell you whether or not the fish was farmed.

Q: What is your take on alpha-lipoic acid?

A: Alpha-lipoic acid (ALA) has a number of admirable qualities including the unique ability to work nearly anywhere in the body. It also appears to be safe, readily converts into a useable form, and neutralizes many different kinds of free radicals. This tiny molecule recycles antioxidants such as vitamin C and E, prolonging their effectiveness.

Terms and definitions

AEROBIC EXERCISE

Prolonged, moderate-intensity work that uses up oxygen at or below the level at which your cardiorespiratory (heart-lung) system can replenish oxygen in the working muscles. Aerobic literally means with oxygen, and it is the only type of exercise, which burns body fat to meet its energy needs. Bodybuilders engage in aerobic workouts to develop additional cardiorespiratory fitness, as well as to burn off excess body fat to achieve peak contest muscularity. Common aerobic activities include running, cycling, swimming, dancing, and walking. Depending on how vigorously you play them, most racquet sports can also be aerobic exercise.

———

ANABOLIC DRUGS

Also called anabolic steroids, these are artificial male hormones that aid in nitrogen retention and thereby add to a male bodybuilder's muscle mass and strength. These drugs are not without hazardous side effects, however, and they are legally available only through a physician's prescription. Steroids are available in most gyms via the black market, but it is very dangerous to use such unknown substances to increase muscle mass.

———

ANAEROBIC EXERCISE

Exercise of much higher intensity than aerobic work, which uses up oxygen more quickly than the body, can replenish it in the working muscles. Anaerobic exercise eventually builds up a significant oxygen debt that forces an athlete to terminate the exercise session rather quickly. Anaerobic exercise, the kind of exercise to which bodybuilding training belongs, burns up glycogen (muscle sugar) to supply its energy needs. Fast sprinting is a typical anaerobic form of exercise.

———

ANDROGENIC DRUGS

Androgenics are drugs that simulate the effects of the male hormone testosterone in the human body. Androgens do build a degree of strength and muscle mass, but they also stimulate secondary sex characteristics such as increased body hair, a deepened voice, and high levels of aggression. Indeed, many bodybuilders and power lifters take androgen to stimulate aggressiveness in the by resulting in more productive workouts.

———

BALANCE

A term referring to an even relationship of body proportions in a man's physique. Perfectly balanced physical proportions are in a much-sought-after trait among competitive bodybuilders.

———

BAR

This is the steel shaft that forms the basic part of barbell or dumbbell. These bars are normally about one inch thick, and they are often encased in a revolving metal sleeve.

———

BARBELL

Normally measuring between four and seven feet in length, a barbell is the most basic piece of weight-training and bodybuilding equipment. Indeed, you can train every major skeletal muscle group in your body using on a barbell. There are two major and types of barbells used for exercise in common use, adjustable sets; in which you can easily add or subtract plates by removing a detachable outside collar held in place on each side by a set screw. And fixed barbells; in which the plates are either welded or bolted permanently in place. Fixed weights are arranged in variety poundages on long racks in commercial bodybuilding gyms, the approximate poundage for each one painted or etched on the bar. Fixed weights relieve you of the problem of changing plates on your barbell for each new exercise. While fixed barbells and dumbbells are normally found in large commercial gyms, adjustable barbell and dumbbell sets are more frequently used at home.

———

BASIC EXERCISE

This is a bodybuilding exercise, which stresses the largest muscle groups of your body (e.g., the thighs, back, and/or chest), often in combination with smaller muscles. You will be able to use very heavy weights in basic exercises in order to build great muscle mass and physical power. Typical basic movements include squats, bench presses, and deadlifts.

———

BENCHES

A wide variety of exercise benches is available for use in doing barbell and dumbbell exercises either lying or seated on a bench. The most common type of bench, a flat exercise bench, can be used for chest, shoulder, and arm movements. Incline and decline benches (which are angled at about 30-45 degrees) allow movements for the chest, shoulder, and arms.

———

BIOMECHANICS

The scientific study of body positions, or form, in sport. In bodybuilding, biomechanics studies body form when exercising with weights. When you have good biomechanics in a bodybuilding exercise, you will be safely placing maximum beneficial stress on your working muscles.

———

BMR

The basal metabolic rate is the speed at which your resting body burns calories to provide for its basic survival needs. You can elevate your BMR and more easily achieve lean body mass through consistent exercise, and particularly through aerobic workouts.

———

BODYBUILDING

A type of weight training applied in conjunction with sound nutritional practices to alter the shape of one's body. In the context of this book, bodybuilding is a competitive sport nationally and internationally in both amateur and professional categories for men, women, and mixed pairs. However, a majority of individuals uses bodybuilding methods merely to lose excess body fat or build up a too thin part of the body.

———

BURN

This is a burning sensation that you feel in the muscle that you are training. This burn is caused by a rapid buildup of fatigue toxins in the muscle and is a good indication that you are optimally working a muscle group. The best bodybuilders consistently forge past the pain barrier erected by muscle burn and consequently build very massive, highly defined muscle.

———

BURNS

A training technique used to push a set past the normal failure point, and thereby to stimulate it to greater hypertrophy. Burns consist of short, quick, bouncy reps 2-4 inches in range of motion. Most bodybuilders do 8-12 burns at the end of a set that has already been taken to failure. They generate terrific burn in the muscles, hence the name of this technique.

———

CARDIORESPIRATORY FITNESS

This is the physical fitness condition of the heart, circulatory system and lungs that is indicative of good aerobic fitness.

———

CHEATING

A method of pushing a muscle to keep working far past the point at which it would normally fail to continue contracting due to excessive fatigue buildup. In cheating you will use a self-administered body swing, jerk, or otherwise poor exercise form once you have reached the failure point to take some of the pressure off the muscles and allow them to continue a set for two or three repetitions past failure.

———

CHINNING BAR

A bar attached high on the wall or gym ceiling, on which you can do chins, hanging leg raises, and other movements for your upper body. A chinning bar is analogous to the high bar male gymnasts use in national and international competitions.

____

CIRCUIT TRAINING

A special form of bodybuilding through which you can simultaneously increase aerobic conditioning, muscle mass, and strength. In circuit training, you will plan a series of 10-20 exercises in a circuit around the gym. The exercises chosen should stress all parts of the body. These movements are performed with an absolute minimum of rest between exercises. Then at the end of a circuit, a rest interval of 2-5 minutes is taken before going through the circuit again. Three-five circuits would constitute a circuit-training program.

____

CLEAN

This movement consists of raising a barbell or two dumbbells from the floor to your shoulders in one smooth motion to prepare for an overhead lift. To properly execute a clean movement, you must use the coordinated strength of your legs, back, shoulders, and arms.

____

COLLAR

A clamp is used to hold plates securely in place on a barbell or dumbbell bar. The cylindrical metal clamps are held in place on the bar by means of a setscrew threaded through the collar and tightened securely against the bar. Inside collars keep plates from sliding inward and injuring your hands, while outside collars keep plates from sliding off the barbell in the middle of an exercise.

____

CUT UP (OR CUT)

A term used to denote a bodybuilder who has an extremely high degree of muscular definition due to a low degree of body fat.

____

DEFINITION

The absence of fat over clearly delineated muscular movement. Definition is often referred to as "muscularity," and a highly defined bodybuilder has so little body fat that very fine grooves of muscularity called "striations" will be clearly visible over each major muscle group.

____

DENSITY

This is the hardness of the muscle, which is also related to muscular definition. A bodybuilder can be well defined and still have excess fat within each major muscle complex. However, when he has muscle density, even this intramuscular fat has been eliminated. A combination of muscle mass and muscle density is highly prized among all competitive bodybuilders.

———

DIPPING BAR

Parallel bars set high enough above the floor to allow you to do dips between them, leg raises for your abdominal, and a variety of other exercises. Some gyms have dipping bars, which are angled inward at one end; these can be used when changing your grip width on dips.

———

DIURETICS

Sometimes called "water pills," these drugs and herbal preparations remove excess water from bodybuilder's system just prior to a show. This reveals greater muscular detail. Harsh chemical diuretics can be quite harmful to your health, particularly if they are used on a chronic basis. Two of the side effects of excessive chemical diuretic use are muscle cramps and heart arrhythmias (irregular heart beats).

———

DUMBBELL

Essentially, a dumbbell is a short-handled barbell (usually 10-16 inches in length) intended primarily for use with one in each hand. Dumbbells are especially valuable when training the arms and shoulders, but can be used to build up almost any muscles.

———

EXERCISE

Movements such as a seated pulley row, barbell curl, bench press, or seated calf raise, etc that you perform in your workouts.

———

EZ-CURL BAR

A special type of barbell used in many arm exercises, but particularly for standing EZ-bar curls wherein it removes strain from your wrists. An EX-curl bar is also occasionally called a "cambered bar." Albert Beckles, one of the sport's most successful professionals from the 1980's, whimsically calls this piece of equipment a "wiggly bar" because of its shape.

———

FAILURE

That point in an exercise, which you have fully fatigued your working muscles. They can no longer complete an additional repetition of a movement with strict biomechanics. You should always take your post-warm-up sets at least to the point of momentary muscular failure, and frequently past that point.

———

FLEXIBILITY

A suppleness of joints, muscle masses, and connective tissues, which lets you, move your limbs over an exaggerated range of motion, a valuable quality in bodybuilding training, since it promotes optimum physical development. Flexibility can only be attained through systematic stretching training, which should form a cornerstone of your overall bodybuilding philosophy.

———

FORCED REPS

Forced reps are a frequently used method of extending a set past the point of failure to induce greater gains in muscle mass and quality. With forced reps, a training partner pulls upward on the bar just enough for you to grind out two or three reps past the failure threshold.

———

FORM

This is simply another word to indicate the biomechanics used during the performance of any bodybuilding or weight-training movement. Perfect form involves moving only the muscles specified in an exercise description, while moving the weight over the fullest possible range of motion.

———

FREE WEIGHTS

Equipment such as: Barbells, dumbbells, and related equipment. Serious bodybuilders use a combination of free weights and such exercise machines as those manufactured by Nautilus and Universal Gyms, but they primarily use free weights in their workouts.

———

GIANT SETS

Performing a series of 3-5 exercises, done with little or no rest between each movements, and a rest interval of 3-4 minutes between each giant sets. You can perform giant sets for either two antagonistic muscle groups or a single body part.

———

HYPERTROPHY

This means increase in muscle mass and an improvement in relative muscular strength. Placing an "over-load" on the working muscles with various training techniques during a bodybuilding workout induces hypertrophy.

———

IFBB

The International Federation of Bodybuilders, the gigantic sports federation founded in1946 by Joe and Ben Weider. With more than 120 member nations, the IFBB proves that bodybuilding is one of the most popular of all sports on the international level.

Through its member national federations, the IFBB oversees competitions in each nation, and it directly administers amateur and professional competition for men, women, and mixed pairs internationally.

———

INTENSITY

The degree of effort that you put into each set of your workout. The more intensity you place on a working muscle, the more quickly it will increase in hypertrophy. The most basic methods of increasing intensity are to use heavier weights in good form in each exercise, do more reps with a set weight, or perform a consistent number of sets and reps with a particular weight in a movement, but progressively reducing the length of rest intervals between sets.

———

ISOLATION EXERCISE

In contrast to a basic exercise, an isolation movement stresses a single muscle group (or sometimes just part of a single muscle) in relative isolation from the remainder of the body. Isolation exercises are good for shaping and defining various muscle groups. For your thighs: squats would be a typical basic movement. While leg extensions would be the equivalent isolation exercise.

———

JUICE

A slang term for anabolic steroids, e.g., being "on the juice."

———

LAYOFF

Most intelligent bodybuilders take a one or two-week layoff from bodybuilding training from time to time, during which they totally avoid the gym. A layoff after a period of intense pre-competition preparation is particularly beneficial as a means of allowing the body to completely rest, recuperate, and heal any minor training injuries that might have cropped up.

———

LIFTING BELT

This is a leather belt 3-5 inches wide at the back that is fastened tightly around your waist when you do squats, heavy back work, and overhead pressing movements. A lifting belt adds stability to your midsection, preventing lower back and abdominal injuries.

———

MASS

The size of the entire physique or the size of each muscle group. As long as you also have a high degree of muscularity and good balance of physical proportions, muscle mass is a highly prized quality among competitive bodybuilders.

MUSCULARITY

An alternative term for "definition" or "cuts."

NPC

The National Physique Committee Inc., which administers men's and women's amateur bodybuilding competitions in the United States. The NPC National Champions in each weight division are annually sent abroad to compete in the IFBB World Championships.

NUTRITION

The applied science of eating to foster greater health, fitness, and muscular grains. Through correct application of nutritional practices, you can selectively add muscle mass to your physique, or totally strip away all body fat, revealing the hard-earned muscles lying beneath your skin.

OLYMPIC BARBELL

A special type of barbell used in weightlifting and powerlifting competitions, but also used by bodybuilders in heavy basic exercises such as squats, bench presses, barbell be rows, standing barbell curls, standing barbell presses, and deadlifts. An Olympic barbell sans collars weighs 45 pounds, and each collar weighs five pounds.

OLYMPIC LIFTING

The type of weightlifting competition contested at the Olympic Games every four years, as well as at national and international competitions each year. Two lifts (the snatch and the clean jerk) are contested in a wide variety of weight classes.

OVERLOAD

The amount of weight that you force a muscle to use that is over and above its normal strength ability. Applying an overload to a muscle forces it to increase in hypertrophy.

PEAK

The absolute zenith of competitive condition achieved by a bodybuilder. To peak out optimally for a bodybuilding show, you must intelligently combine bodybuilding training, aerobic workouts, diet, mental conditioning, tanning, and a large number of other preparatory factors.

PLATES

The flat discs placed on the ends of barbell and dumbbell bars to increase the weight of the apparatus. Although some plates are made from vinyl-covered concrete, the best and most durable plates are manufactured from metal. Plates range in size from 1.25 - 100 pounds but using the term "plate" by itself refers to the 45 pounders.

———

POSE

Each individual stance that a bodybuilder does onstage in order to highlight his muscular development.

———

POUNDAGE

The amount of weight that you use in an exercise, whether that weight is on a barbell, dumbbell, or exercise machine.

———

POWER LIFTING

A second form of competitive weightlifting (not contested in the Olympics, however) featuring three lifts: The squat, bench press, and deadlift. Power lifting is contested both nationally and internationally in a wide variety of weight classes for both men and women.

———

PROGRESSION

The act of gradually adding to the amount of resistance that you use in each exercise. Without consistent progression in your workouts, you won't overload your muscles sufficiently to promote optimum increases in hypertrophy.

———

PUMP

The tight, blood-congested feeling in a muscle after it has been intensely trained. Muscle pump is caused by a rapid influx of blood into the muscles to remove fatigue toxins and replace supplies of fuel and oxygen. A good muscle pump is one of the indicators that show you have optimally worked a muscle group.

———

REPETITION (REP)

Each individual count of an exercise that is performed. Series of repetitions called "sets" are performed on each exercise in your training program.

———

RESISTANCE

The actual amount of weight that you are using in any exercise.

———

REST INTERVAL

The brief rest between sets that allows your body to partially recuperate prior to initiating the succeeding set. Usually between 1-5 minutes depending on how big the muscle group is.

———

RIPPED

The same as cut up.

———

ROUTINE

Also called a training schedule or program, a routine is the total list of exercise, sets, and reps (and sometimes weights) used in one training session.

———

SET

A grouping of repetitions that is followed by a rest interval and usually another set. Three to five sets are usually performed of each exercise.

———

SLEEVE

The hollow metal tube fit over the bar on most exercise barbell and dumbbell sets. This sleeve makes it easier for the bar to rotate in your hands as you do an exercise.

———

SPOTTERS

Training partners who stand by to act as safety helpers when you perform such heavy exercises as squats and bench presses. If you are stuck under and weight or begin to lose control of it, spotters can rescue you and prevent needless injuries.

———

STEROIDS

Prescription drugs which mimic male hormones, but without most of the androgenic side effects of actual testosterone. Many bodybuilders use these drugs to help increase muscle mass and strength.

———

STICKING POINT

A stalling out of bodybuilding progress. Also called a plateau.

———

STRETCHING

A type of exercise program in which you assume exaggerated postures that stretch muscles, joints, and connective tissues, hold these positions for several seconds, relax and then repeat the postures. Regular stretching exercise promotes body flexibility.

———

STRETCH MARKS

Tiny tears in a bodybuilder's skin caused by poor diet and in addition, rapid increases in bodyweight. If you notice stretch marks forming on your own body (usually around your pectoral-deltoid tie-ins), rub vitamin E cream over them two or three times per day, and try cutting back on your body weight by reducing body fat levels.

———

STRIATIONS

The tiny grooves of muscle across major muscle groups in a highly defined bodybuilder.

———

SUPERSETS

Series of two exercises performed with no rest between sets and a normal rest interval between supersets. Supersets increase training intensity by reducing the average length of rest interval between sets. They are also performed on the same muscle, not two different muscle groups.

———

SUPPLEMENTS

Concentrated vitamins, minerals, and proteins used by bodybuilders to improve the overall quality of their diets. Many bodybuilders believe that food supplements help to promote quality muscle growth.

———

SYMMETRY

The shape or general outline of a person's body, as when seen in silhouette. If you have good symmetry, you will have relatively wide shoulders, flaring lats, a small waist-hip structure, and generally small joints.

———

TESTOSTERONE

The male hormone primarily responsible for the maintenance of muscle mass and strength induced by heavy training. Testosterone is secondarily responsible for developing such secondary male sex characteristics as a deep voice, body hair, and male pattern baldness.

———

TRISETS

Series of three exercises performed with no rest between movements and a normal rest interval between trisets. Trisets increase training intensity by reducing the average length of rest interval between sets.

––––––––

VASCULARITY

A prominence of veins and arteries over the muscles and beneath the skin of a sell-defined bodybuilder.

––––––––

WARM-UP

The 5-15 minutes session of light calisthenics, aerobic exercise, and stretching taken prior to handling heavy bodybuilding training movements. A good warm-up helps to prevent injuries and actually allows you to get more out of your training than if you went into a workout cold.

––––––––

WEIGHT

The same as Poundage or Resistance.

––––––––

WEIGHTLIFTING

The competitive form of weight training in which each athlete attempts to lift as much as he can in well-defined exercises. Olympic lifting and power lifting are the two types of weightlifting competition.

––––––––

WEIGHT TRAINING

An umbrella term used to categorize all acts of using resistance training. Weight training can be used to improve the body, rehabilitate injuries, improve sports conditioning, or as a competitive activity in terms of bodybuilding weightlifting.

––––––––

WORKOUT

A bodybuilding or weight-training session.

###